Women & Diabetes

Life Planning

for Health

and Wellness

By Laurinda M. Poirier, RN, MPH, CDE
& Katharine M. Coburn, MPH

▲.American Diabetes Association.

Book Acquisitions	Susan Reynolds
Editor	Sherrye Landrum
Cover Design	Wickham & Associates, Inc.
Illustrations	Odette Brown
Desktop Publishing	Insight Graphics
Production Director	Carolyn R. Segree
Production Coordinator	Peggy M. Rote

The suggestions and information contained in this publication are generally consistent with the *Clinical Practice Recommendations* and other policies of the American Diabetes Association, but they do not represent the policy or position of the Association or any of its boards or committees. Reasonable steps have been taken to ensure the accuracy of the information presented. However, the American Diabetes Association cannot ensure the safety or efficacy of any product or service described in this publication. Individuals are advised to consult a physician or other appropriate health care professional before undertaking any diet or exercise program or taking any medication referred to in this publication. Professionals must use and apply their own professional judgment, experience, and training and should not rely solely on the information contained in this publication before prescribing any diet, exercise, or medication. The American Diabetes Association—its officers, directors, employees, volunteers, and members—assumes no responsibility or liability for personal or other injury, loss, or damage that may result from the suggestions or information in this publication.

Printed in the United States of America

American Diabetes Association, Inc.
1660 Duke Street
Alexandria, VA 22314

Library of Congress Cataloging-in-Publication Data

Poirier, Laurinda M., 1960–
    Women & diabetes: life planning for health and wellness / by Laurinda M. Poirier & Katharine M. Coburn.
        p.   cm.
    Includes bibliographical references.
    ISBN 0-945448-77-5 (pbk.)
    1. Diabetes--Popular works.   2. Women--Diseases.   3. Women--Health and hygiene.   I. Coburn, Katharine M., 1962–   .   II. Title.
RC660.4.P65   1997
616.4'62'082--dc21   97–3159
                                                                                    CIP

Dedication

In memory of my sister Leetha Poirier Trainor whose life experiences and challenges continue to feed my passion for helping women to find their voices.

To my parents, Jeanne and Donald Poirier, for their strength and inspiration.

—LMP

To my husband, Kevin Coburn, and our sons, Donald and Miles, for being there for me.

—KMC

To all the women who have taught us, and still teach us, about the realities of living with a chronic disease.

Our deepest appreciation goes to Dorothea F. Sims whose mentoring showed us that being well depends on the perspective to be gained in befriending diabetes and meeting life's challenges with optimism and grace.

Table of Contents

Preface

This book is for all women who live with the chronic disease, diabetes—young and old, type 1 and type 2, insulin users and non-insulin users. This is also for their loved ones who live and experience the struggles with them and for their health care providers who work beside them on their quest for wellness.

This book is written in honor of the woman with diabetes and for

her *story* and learning along the way,

her *joy* and *zest* for living,

her *desire* to feel whole, beautiful, and valued,

her *tears* that are the jewels of healing,

her *pain* and *fear* of the real and the imagined,

her *spirit* that is tender and giving, and

her *dreams* for a better tomorrow.

As women seek to enhance their sense of well-being, they encounter obstacles along the way. The most common is a general sense of dissatisfaction with who we are, the way we look, and what we do. The challenge to overcome this is universal and unites women of different ages, colors, races, and religions.

We view this book as a send-off, a bon voyage present. It does not make decisions for any of you but illustrates useful perspectives and strategies that may help you determine what you need, make decisions for your own wellness, and grow.

We express our gratitude to the women who personalized the messages in this book with their voices of reality: Deanna Kredenser, Margaret Lawlor, Lynn Fischhaber, and Dorothy DeMatteo.

A special thanks to Elizabeth C. Bashoff, MD, at the Joslin Diabetes Center, for her critiques along the way.

We thank Josie McKee and Allyson Coburn for their courageous ways of meeting their health challenges. They revealed to us how a woman mobilizes power when she chooses to respond to her challenges by growing through the experience. Their examples enrich so many lives.

And finally (for her wisdom and support), we thank our editor, Sherrye Landrum, who made this possible.

About the Authors

Through my work as a diabetes nurse educator at the Joslin Diabetes Center and Dartmouth-Hitchcock Medical Center, I have learned about the unique challenges of living with diabetes and the creative ways people respond to these challenges. I have grown to appreciate how diabetes colors women's dreams and realities. I have seen the healing power in women bonding together. My commitment to helping women with diabetes grew after I witnessed the sense of isolation experienced by many of the women I worked with in New Hampshire and Vermont. Their quest to be heard, valued, and strengthened motivated me to develop a one-day workshop that enabled them to share their stories and learn from each other. Their stories and those of my own family fueled my interest in helping women find their strengths and discover their voices.

Committing yourself to wellness is no easy task. In my personal quest, I have become aware of my own vulnerabilities and struggles with time demands, self-image, and healthy behaviors. This awareness motivates me to share the insights and strategies that I have learned from my own experience and from the experiences of other women.

—*Laurinda M. Poirier*

I was diagnosed with diabetes as a young child. Attending teaching clinics and diabetes camp helped me learn to manage and accept having diabetes. As I grew up, I became interested in how to make life better for people with diabetes. I developed diabetes education programs and served on the boards of the ADA New Hampshire Affiliate and the ADA Vermont Affiliate. I learned to appreciate the power of supportive people in assisting others to lead healthy, enriched lives.

My adventures as a woman with diabetes have shaped my personal and professional career paths. I have always led my life to the fullest and sought to enable others to do the same, regardless of their past or present circumstances.

As the coordinator of the Community Health Education Section of the Center for Continuing Education at Dartmouth-Hitchcock Medical Center, I work with health care providers, community organizations, and employers to promote individual health through education. I also work at Dartmouth Medical School facilitating service-learning opportunities that teach medical students to be responsive to patient needs. Personally and professionally, I am optimistic that providers will empower women with diabetes and inspire them to lead fulfilled lives.

—*Katharine M. Coburn*

Struggle

A man found a cocoon of the Emperor moth and took it home to watch it emerge. One day a small opening appeared, and for several hours the moth struggled but couldn't seem to force its body past a certain point.

Deciding something was wrong, the man took scissors and snipped the remaining bit of cocoon. The moth emerged easily, its body large and swollen, the wings small and shriveled.

He expected that in a few hours the wings would spread out in their natural beauty, but they did not. Instead of developing into a creature free to fly, the moth spent its life dragging around a swollen body and shriveled wings.

The constricting cocoon and the struggle necessary to pass through the tiny opening are God's way of forcing fluid from the body into the wings. The "merciful" snip was, in reality, cruel. Sometimes the struggle is exactly what we need.

—Jason Elias and Katherine Ketcham
In the House of the Moon: Reclaiming the Feminine Spirit of Healing

Chapter 1

My Own Reality: Who Am I as a Woman With Diabetes?

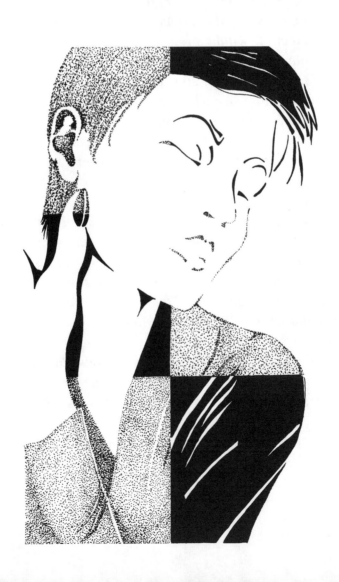

The Circle

All is a circle within me.
> *I am ten thousand winters old.*
> *I am as young as a newborn flower.*
> *I am a buffalo in its grave.*
> *I am a tree in bloom.*

All is a circle within me.
> *I have seen the world through an eagle's eyes.*
> *I have seen it from a gopher's hole.*
> *I have seen the world on fire*
> *And the sky without a moon.*

All is a circle within me.
> *I have gone into the earth and out again.*
> *I have gone to the edge of the sky.*

Now all is at peace within me.
Now all has a place to come home.

> —Nancy Wood
> *Spirit Walker*

Anna was striking. At 72, she was radiant and beautiful despite the wrinkles, the dependency on a wheelchair for mobility, and even the recent loss of a grandchild. Her tenderness and comfort with herself radiated to others beyond the cloak of an aging body. She did not dwell on the fact that she was unable to keep up with the rest of the group nor that she needed help with some of her diabetes self-care tasks. Her focus was on living the moment, enjoying the view, and experiencing a new adventure. Her acceptance of herself enabled her to go beyond any external limitations and events imposed on her.

It is possible to live a rewarding life as a woman with diabetes and to feel whole and fulfilled. Women like Anna remind us that our state of wellness is determined by much more than the absence of illness. "Well" people can have debilitating health conditions. Wellness is a state of feeling good about yourself. That means you not only surrender to but honor who you are, even the part of yourself that is ill. Wellness defined this way honors the whole person and does not depend on the illness going away.

Diabetes is a chronic illness—it never goes away. It becomes part of you, like the color of your eyes. It will be your companion, and it will be your teacher, too. Learning to live well with diabetes is like having a lifetime job. Like any job, this one involves learning about your limits, your potential for change, as well as your physical and emotional needs. It involves being able to make a promise to yourself and keeping it. Living well with diabetes is not as simple as taking the right medication at the right time, eating the right amount of food, or exercising! As you know, you also need to be flexible and to adapt to the unexpected. Whether you have type 1 or type 2, diabetes is something you'll think about every day. What you think will affect what you do and how well you feel.

To begin with, if you have not taken care of yourself or your diabetes in the past, do not waste energy now on regret or guilt. This is a poor investment of your precious time and energy. Acknowledge and respect the path that you have traveled this far and begin to explore how you can make a difference now. Look at the big picture. Consider what you want out of life as a woman who also happens to have diabetes. How do you want your life with diabetes to change?

This moment in your life is an opportunity to think about the future, to set new life goals, and to decide how to reach them. Everyone needs time for reflection and renewal. This is what teachers do on sabbaticals and business people do during a retreat. This is the time to fuel your imagination, to be creative, to have some fun, and to return to your life as a woman with diabetes in new ways that feel good to you.

Most women want to do what is best for themselves, but knowing what is best and how to do it are not always clear. With diabetes there are no real milestones, so you may feel like you endlessly seek without arriving. When you consider managing diabetes as a career, you see your challenge in a different light. With this job, as with every job, comes a set of rights, responsibilities, and pressures as well as opportunities to grow. It requires you to be motivated and flexible, to manage stress, and to solve problems. This job will teach you about yourself and help you improve your self image, if you let it.

Perfection: Is It Possible?

We all feel the pressure to be "superwoman" at different points in our lives. Yet, it is never clear how Superwoman can do all that is expected. If you are trying to live up to images of the perfect woman or the perfect woman with diabetes, you may make yourself crazy trying to juggle all the demands of self-care, home, and work life. You may be trying to do the impossible. Every woman needs realistic responsibilities and realistic expectations of what she can accomplish.

By whose standards do you judge yourself? Our society tends to value women who are slim, successful, and wealthy. Do you try to mold yourself to these criteria, disregarding your own abilities and individuality? In the same way, do you just accept the health goals set by your diabetes care provider? If you don't participate in setting your goals, you begin to define your sense of worth by external measures like the numbers on your meter or the pounds you lose. But by these standards, perfection is not possible, especially when you are managing a chronic disease. Focusing on perfection limits your satisfaction with your life.

Your job requires you to listen to your body and to take time to care for yourself. These are good and powerful things to learn to do. But diabetes care is often demanding with few immediate or visible rewards. The thoughts and ideas in this book are based on the experiences of other women with diabetes and provide you an opportunity to understand your own experience with new appreciation and tenderness.

This is the time to stop judging your actions as good or bad, success or failure. It is a time to let go of the guilt that you cannot be everything to everyone, that you cannot be perfect. No one can. This will be the beginning of your wisdom. Women are by nature, healers. You will heal when you are true to yourself, begin to feel your wholeness, and listen to your own spirit. This is a job that you can do.

My Partnership With Diabetes

As a woman with diabetes, you have the "job" of living in partnership with this aspect of yourself. To succeed in your career as a manager of diabetes, you have to develop a healthy relationship with yourself and your disease. How do you regard your diabetes? Is it a failure or a character flaw, something to be ashamed of or to hide? Do you think it detracts from your value as a woman? Is diabetes the enemy that drains you emotionally or physically, a dragon to fight and slay? Or is it a part of you that you accept and care for?

Each of us wants to be a whole woman whose life is full and balanced. To do that, we must recognize all the parts of ourselves and fit them together. How would you describe yourself? Imagine that the circle below represents you, a whole person. Where would you place diabetes—inside or outside the circle? Take a moment to write the word *diabetes* where it fits best for you.

YOU

Now, write in the words or qualities that describe other parts of you, your passions, likes, and strengths. Did you say that you are a painter, a cook, a mother, a gardener? Or did you note your passion for quilting, reading, or traveling? How did diabetes come into the picture? Examine your circle again. How much energy do you give to each part of you? How much is your physical health the focus of your life?

Let's examine how some other women have completed the circle. Which response rings true for you?

"Diabetes does not exist!"   *"Diabetes is my life!"*

Diabetes (**Life**)   (**Diabetes**) **Life**

"Diabetes is a part of me."

(**Life & Diabetes**)

Diabetes does not exist!

Susan wakes every morning, takes her medication, and puts her diabetes away for the rest of the day.

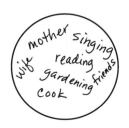

Diabetes

Note that for Susan, diabetes is placed outside of the circle. It is separate from her definition of self. She denies the presence of diabetes, lives life, and makes choices without regard to how diabetes fits into the picture. Diabetes is the enemy, somehow, and is only dealt with when there is a problem. Statements like "I don't have time for diabetes;" "I will not let it control me;" "It will not get in the way;" are used often by women who share Susan's view of diabetes. Words like fight, flaw, anger, fear, and resentment reflect their attitudes and emotions.

Let's consider what happens when Susan treats her diabetes as separate from herself or as something bad. Refusing to acknowledge the importance of diabetes can lead to poor diabetes control, which puts Susan at risk for other health problems. She may experience many low blood sugars that spoil her daily plans or high blood sugars that make her feel sluggish and ill. Susan may be putting herself at risk for diabetes complications such as eye disease or nerve damage.

When Susan refuses to do diabetes tasks or approaches them with resentment, she is feeding herself with negative and unhealthy messages. Over time this dissatisfaction with this part of herself will create "dis"ease and imbalance. Denial builds stress and takes energy to maintain. In a sense, Susan is trying to quit a job that she has inherited for life. It can't be done.

Why do women like Susan regard the diabetes part of themselves so negatively? Having diabetes makes her feel different. She feels that she is not accepted by her peers, family, or society. It is difficult for people without diabetes to understand why she must eat a certain way or do special things for herself. High and low blood sugars complicate things even further. Others may look at the strong emotions that accompany swings in blood sugar, like anger or crying, as exaggerated or done to get attention. It is often difficult to take time from group activities to treat low blood sugar or to recover from its impact. Susan may feel the need to overcompensate for the fact that diabetes got in the way, or she may feel ashamed. Considering this very common scenario, it is no surprise that Susan regards her diabetes as something bad and unwanted! She is being forced to change, and she's fighting it.

Women often feel by their own standards (or society's) that they should keep quiet about their own needs. Society seems to have little patience for people who are different or who focus on themselves. This makes it that much more difficult to pay attention to diabetes and health needs.

Diabetes is my life!

Emma, who has type 2 diabetes, often refuses to join her friends at the bridge club in order to be home to check her blood sugar and eat her meal on time.

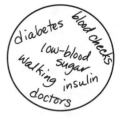

Jennifer, with type 1 diabetes, works out every day after work, refuses to eat out with friends for fear of having to eat foods not on her meal plan, and checks her blood sugar five to ten times a day with the hopes of keeping them between 70–130 mg/dl. She is skeptical of dating because she feels that a prospective partner will think diabetes is a burden.

Women like Emma and Jennifer define whatever they do or are capable of doing by their diabetes. Diabetes is the major focus of their existence. Developing or creating healthy relationships with others, going to social functions, taking a job, having children, and even accepting spontaneous invitations are all limited by diabetes. Emma and Jennifer spend all their energy thinking about what to eat, how and when to exercise, and looking out for the next hypoglycemic episode. Jennifer's sense of worth is defined by whether or not her blood sugars are within target. When they are not, she is miserable. She exercises more, eats less, and checks her blood sugar more often. Diabetes has become her life. Her life is not balanced; it is not full.

How do women get into this trap? Diabetes is complex. Keeping track of blood sugar levels, making treatment decisions, and responding to high and low blood sugars can easily consume your energy! You could spend a great deal of time trying to figure out why your blood sugar fluctuates and dealing with the emotional baggage like frustration and guilt that comes with the highs and lows. Relax a little and realize that you can't figure out each and every number. It truly is impossible, so don't make yourself crazy trying.

Motivated to be healthy by fear of complications, Emma and Jennifer try every moment of the day to achieve their health goals.

Perhaps they do not understand how changes in food, activity, hormone levels, medications, or hectic schedules can affect their blood sugar, so all they can do is feel guilty when the blood sugars are outside the desired range. They need to know what else they can do. They should know that 20–30% of these values can never be explained, so they won't feel hopeless and helpless. It seems to be easier to turn down the invitation for dinner or let that new relationship go away than to deal with the fluctuations in blood sugar.

Emma and Jennifer's lives are dominated by diabetes for good reasons. Diabetes research and health care providers tell you to focus on glucose levels. An important national study proved that keeping blood glucose as close to normal as possible reduces the risk for developing complications! Now, that is a big reason to keep diabetes in the front of your mind! Due to time constraints during a routine office visit, health care providers may tend to focus on your glucose levels or your success in achieving other treatment goals. This focus only reinforces Emma's and Jennifer's unhealthy preoccupation with their blood sugar. And it leaves all the other ways to measure success unexplained and unexplored. Even though your provider may not have the time to pay attention to how you are challenged emotionally by diabetes, it is an important aspect of your self-care. You may need to seek out other resources to help you.

What about you?

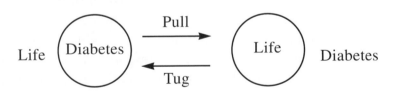

Many women find themselves going back and forth between these two ways of relating to their diabetes. At one point it dominates their life; at another, it is ignored. This is normal. Expect it. However, if you get stuck in one of these ways of relating to your diabetes for long periods of time, you're out of balance and will face unhealthy emotional and physical consequences.

Now let's consider how diabetes, or any chronic health problem, can become a healthy part of your life. You can learn how to pay attention to your diabetes and still keep it in a healthy balance with the rest of your life. Diabetes can be simply one aspect of your life that requires periodic attention and work.

Imagine the circle again with your diabetes in a positive light.

Diabetes is part of me!

Brenda is a mom and a grandmother, with a part-time job and a home to maintain. She takes diabetes pills twice a day and monitors her glucose levels one to three times a day. She has learned to count carbohydrates and to adjust her food intake to fit in hiking with her family, dining out with friends, and biking.

Rebecca, 32, manages her diabetes with an insulin pump. She is constantly making decisions and trying to avoid hypoglycemia. She is a waitress and graduate student. She works hard at including time for relaxation and cross country skiing.

Brenda treats diabetes as a priority along with other activities that she cares about. Diabetes does not carry a good or bad label. It is just there. When it needs attention, she provides it, not with resentment but with caring. Because she respects diabetes as a part of her, she accepts that it will periodically challenge her. Once the challenge has been addressed, she can refocus her energy on other aspects of her life, such as gardening, child care, or biking. To develop this balanced attitude toward her diabetes, Brenda had to learn a lot about her own body and about diabetes, and she reached out to her family and health care team for support.

Rebecca works equally hard at keeping her diabetes in perspective. At times she finds herself resenting her diabetes because it makes life difficult. But her resentment, even though it is strong, is healthy. She doesn't ignore her diabetes or pretend it isn't there. She accepts it as part of her reality.

Perceptions and Expectations

Fairly early in life, we arrive at an idea about who we are, what we are capable of doing, and how we should live. Sometimes we shortchange ourselves by these definitions or ideas. Instead of guiding us, these images act like a cage, actually preventing us from changing and growing.

> *Ellen has found a hidden ability and passion for long-distance biking. Two years ago, her image of herself was not as an athlete. This self-definition was based on her awkward experiences with baseball and basketball as a child. Letting go of this limited self-image, she participated in a short bike-a-thon and found she enjoyed it. With subsequent bike trips, her enjoyment grew, and she was willing to go greater distances. One day she realized that she did have athletic abilities. They were just different from her preconceived notion of what being "athletic" was. Now, she enjoys this newfound part of herself and has learned that she does not have to bike at a competitive level to express herself in new ways or to have fun.*

So often, women limit their choices and enjoyment because of preconceived ideas or past experiences. Ellen was limited by two ideas. The first was that because she was not good at sports, she was not good at any athletic activity. The second was that she had to be good enough to compete. Releasing herself from these expectations brought her newfound joy! How often do your perceptions about yourself, your diabetes, or your previous experiences limit your potential today?

Feeding Your Soul

*The heart eats food from every companion; the head
receives nourishment from every piece of knowledge.*
—Rumi

You often hear "We are what we eat." In reality who we are is a product of what we feed ourselves on three levels: physical, spiritual, and intellectual. How are you nourished? What messages do you feed yourself? What messages do you accept from others about yourself? What do you do to replenish your emotional and physical stores? Physically, you "replenish" your stores by eating healthfully or getting enough sleep. Feeding your heart and mind requires giving yourself nurturing messages, thinking beautiful thoughts, reading about and learning new things, and seeking encouragement from others who like and enjoy you.

Consider what types of internal messages you accept from yourself or from others. Is there a critic inside you, ready to cut you down, one that actually drains your energy and confidence? Is there a harsh voice or a judge inside you who doubts your abilities? Or do you have an inner coach and cheerleader? Are you guided by a nurturing and encouraging voice that tells you to reach for your dreams? Is there one that comforts you through difficult times? Do you tell yourself how great you are?

Do any of these messages sound familiar to you? Which ones feel more supportive and comfortable?

"I can't do that!" "It isn't good enough!"
"I've tried everything!"
"It is possible." "One thing at a time." "I can do it."
"It is OK to make mistakes."

What we feel and believe about ourselves colors every experience we have. A woman who feels good about herself is likely to cope with the crises in life better than the woman who is fed with negative messages.

Carrie referred to her body as a temple. She was cautious about how much she drank and avoided cigarette smoking. She taught me that our bodies are receptacles that are influenced by what we do and the choices we make. She lived by the belief that if she fed herself in an unhealthy manner or treated her body disrespectfully, it would be much more difficult to be well and to live fully.

What we choose to feed our bodies physically, emotionally, and spiritually is similar to the quality of gas and oil we choose to put into our motor vehicles. If you constantly feed yourself negative or discouraging thoughts, you will find it very difficult to achieve any sense of health and wellness.

Language: The Power of Words

The words we use to describe diabetes and ourselves will influence our experience, too. Medical jargon can be derogatory. Even though many of these terms cannot be avoided, being aware of the words and phrases we use can help us achieve and maintain healthy balance in our lives.

Consider what words you use to talk about diabetes. Reflect on how these words make you feel about yourself as a woman. Look at the phrases below and choose the one that reveals the woman you are. Who lives inside the external cloak you see in the mirror?

I am a diabetic!—No, that isn't right!
I am a person with diabetes!—Yes, but I am more!
I am a woman who happens to have diabetes—That's right but more!
*I am a woman who is in touch with myself
   because of diabetes!*—YEAH!

Consider using the phrase that provides you with a sense of freedom to experience and celebrate yourself in new ways. We hope that you will value the idea that you are not just a diabetic. You are a woman, a person who has diabetes, with your own set of dreams, hopes and desires, unique gifts, and talents.

> *While attending a workshop on health and wellness, Sara learned that she could build a sense of well-being simply by adding the word "honor" to her vocabulary. The trainer in the course used words like honor when talking about a woman's body. Honor. The word alone is sweet, light, and respectful. That word had great impact on how Sara began to think about and care for her own body. She had been used to pushing herself day in and day out until exhaustion forced her to take refuge in sleep. Without meaning to, she had abused her body, taken it for granted, and responded to it only when it was completely exhausted. She had experienced many highs and lows. She did not feel vibrant and energetic. But in the workshop she learned that she should honor her body. When she realized that this is the only body she has and the vehicle that moves her along the journey of life, she embraced the value of treating it better. After the workshop, she was more mindful about the types of food she fed her body, the amount of rest she had, and the ways her blood sugar levels rose and fell.*

Words help give meaning to our experiences. This meaning feeds our beliefs and behavior. By including the word *honor* when speaking or thinking of herself, Sara began to feel better physically and emotionally.

Reshaping Your Outlook

What does it take to regard diabetes as a healthy part of yourself? Honesty. Respect. Courage.

Honesty
- about who you are
- about how you treat and take care of yourself
- about the choices you make
- about what you take for granted and what you ignore

Respect
- your individuality
- that all people make mistakes
- the need to change your approach and attitude

Courage
- to keep looking for truths
- to change

How does diabetes affect you? You experience emotions or physical feelings because of fluctuations in blood sugars that women without diabetes do not. All women feel, at some time, fatigued, irritable, lethargic, or overwhelmed. With diabetes, these feelings may be exaggerated and intense. Your ability to rebound may be a little slower. Most women tend to deny that there is a problem and that the body requires more time to balance itself. Being aware of this will help you give yourself the time you need before you get overwhelmed.

Having diabetes does not make you better or worse then anyone else. It just is part of you. Diabetes is an issue of blood sugars and how food is used by the body. It does not define your value or worth. It is one of the jobs you do. Your challenge will be to accept and to use what diabetes teaches you about yourself.

We invite you to actively participate in directing your life with diabetes instead of passively accepting what may happen. When you play an active role in your own life, you strengthen your sense of integrity. You come to know and then to honor what is right for you. You may not always be able to prevent a health problem or high and low blood sugars, but you can choose how you approach them and how you define your inner self. Who are you, the woman meeting the life challenges today?

Consider developing a healthy relationship with your diabetes, respecting it—not resigning to it—by acknowledging that it is there and needs your attention. In this book, we explore how you can strengthen your ability to manage your life with diabetes. You can learn to listen to your body's needs and how to develop self-care skills.

Chapter 2

My Full-Time Job Managing Diabetes

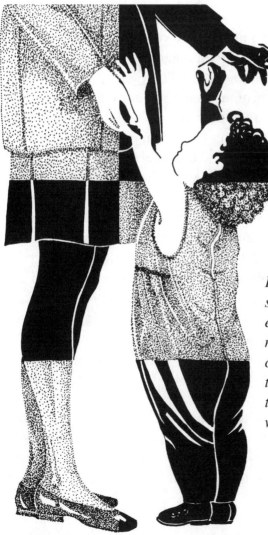

Far away there in the sunshine are my highest aspirations. I may not reach them, but I can look up and see their beauty, believe in them, and try to follow where they lead.
—Louisa May Alcott

Michelle, a woman with diabetes, strives to keep her blood sugar in the target range. Today, she is distressed because only some measurements have been within 80–150 mg/dl for the past two weeks. She is frustrated, weary with effort, and unhappy with the results. Michelle fails to see that over the last two weeks she has had additional pressures from work, a sick loved one to care for, and no time to follow her activity program. She is a woman juggling many demands on her time and energy. It isn't surprising that her glucose control is less than ideal.

Have you ever wondered why you feel exhausted at the end of the day? Or why blood sugar levels do not cooperate with even the best-laid plans? There are good reasons why achieving glucose control, achieving your goals for the day, and maintaining wellness are daily challenges. As a woman, you may juggle multiple demands from work, home, family, as well as take care of yourself. As a woman with diabetes, you also have to integrate all these demands with the daily responsibilities of managing diabetes. Unexpected events and requests from others may periodically distract you from attending to your self-care needs. If left unchecked, these demands can easily consume your energy, leaving you drained and falling short of your life goals.

To help you appreciate all that you do, we would like you to think about managing diabetes as having a full-time job. In fact, it is a life long career of learning who you are, respecting what you find, and honoring what you need. Managing your life and your diabetes with integrity and a sense of self worth calls on your ability to set limits, place yourself high on your list of priorities, and use ongoing training and support.

How aware are you of the demands made on you? How prepared are you to deal with those demands? Through the activities in this chapter, you have the opportunity to see what you do on a daily basis and what you need to do in your job as a manager of diabetes.

Keep a sense of humor as you explore what this job is about and see how expectations of perfection set you up for disappointment and frustration.

Once you know what is asked of you, you can then determine what skills, behaviors, and attitudes you need to help you better deal with the demands of being, first, a woman, and then a woman with diabetes. Knowing is only part of it, however. The next step is committing yourself to action. You must develop and use your skills as well as adopt the behaviors and attitudes that serve you best. This is a challenging career. To help you, you may periodically need to call on your inner coach, that wiser self, to get rid of negative thoughts that sabotage your efforts.

The Job

What is the job of managing life as a woman with diabetes? To help you answer this question, imagine the following want ad showing up in the local newspaper.

WANTED!

Woman to manage life with diabetes, 24 hours a day, 7 days a week, 365 days a year. Requirements include creative skills, flexibility, appreciation for the unexpected, and tolerance for pain. For more details write Box 000.

Asking for more details, you receive the following.

Career Summary

Demanding career involving the use of mental, physical, and technical skills in caring for diabetes and other self-care needs while maintaining home, family and other employment. The responsibilities include, but are not limited to, working in partnership with family and health care providers to develop strategies to manage diabetes and health care needs. Your job is to fit diabetes into your life as a partner, mother, employee, and friend.

All women want a full and balanced life. To reach this goal, a woman must rise to meet many demands, such as interacting with the people who are close to her, meeting the needs of those who depend on her, and ensuring her financial security. These are priorities common to all women. You have an additional responsibility to actively participate in caring for your diabetes and reduce your risks of developing long-term health problems. This job, with all of its complexities, inconveniences, and conflicting demands, has been awarded to you. Let's explore the job requirements.

To give you some insight, let's look at the competing demands that make it difficult for Lucy and Diane to take care of themselves.

Lucy is a single woman. Her job as a graphic artist often requires her to work late and occasionally on weekends. Because she does not rely financially on someone else, she feels pressure to work in a job that will provide her with a certain income and good retirement benefits. She invests a great deal of time going to seminars and taking classes to enhance her career opportunities. Lucy spends her free time helping her sisters take care of her nieces and nephews. She also puts energy into developing and maintaining friendships. Friends operate as family in many situations for support, guidance, and laughter. In between her class and work schedule and connecting with friends and family, Lucy tries to work out at a local club and to take care of her diabetes.

Diane is a wife, a mother of two grown children, and a teacher at the junior high school. She shares the financial and household responsibilities with her husband. She is often tired and drained after dealing with her students. Her days are long, as she grades papers, helps troubled students, and prepares for classes. She is an active member of her church community and joins in running craft fairs and other fundraisers. She and her husband enjoy round-dancing and visiting with their children, who are now in college. She is motivated to work not only for her own satisfaction and personal growth, but also to help support her children in college and pay for the added expense of diabetes supplies.

Lucy and Diane both try to balance all the demands on their time seamlessly. Their unconscious expectation is to do everything well. Their goals include keeping blood sugar levels between 80–150 mg/dl most of the time, keeping their weight stable, and taking care of daily chores, work demands, and family needs without a flaw. They both feel defeated and anxious when things do not go well or when their blood sugars run high.

How realistic are Lucy's and Diane's expectations? Are you like them, trying to be Superwoman and do everything well? Are you aware of all that competes for your time and energy? To fulfill any job, especially this one, it is important to familiarize yourself with what is expected of you on a routine basis—the job expectations. To help you identify these expectations, use the self-assessment at the end of this chapter (pp. 34–38). This assessment outlines the responsibilities commonly required to manage a woman's life and her diabetes. You may be surprised at all that you are already handling!

The Realities of Your Job as Manager of Diabetes

Although perfection is not possible, setting goals and approaching them is the only way you can grow. What are your goals for diabetes and your life? Write them down in the box on the next page.

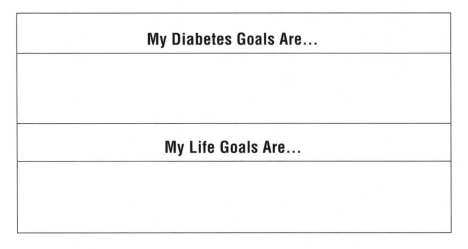

| My Diabetes Goals Are... |
| My Life Goals Are... |

Now, take a moment to reflect on the things you do on a routine basis as a woman with diabetes. Write them down in the box below. Then add to the list below your other responsibilities as a partner, mother, employee, or friend.

| **Diabetes Tasks** |
| The things I need to do to take care of my diabetes include... |
| **Other Tasks** |
| The things I need to do on a routine basis include... |

How do these lists compare to each other? Are they in competition for your time and energy? Do you feel any one area is neglected?

Other women were asked to describe their experience with diabetes. Their responses are listed on the next page. How do they compare to your list? Do you see any to add to your list?

Some women referred to their job as management.

- Time manager
- Manager of blood sugar
- Planner: of meals, social events, self-care, child care
- Stress manager: dealing with my own stress and that of others

Some felt that they were in the business of taking care of others and themselves.

- Caretaker of others: with my needs often overshadowed by the needs of the family
- Troubleshooter: of family disputes as well as those high and low blood sugar levels
- Educator: of others about diabetes and self-care needs
- Doctor: needing to diagnose the major problems to get them attended to properly and quickly
- Dietitian: choosing foods to eat, planning meals, purchasing, and cooking
- Researcher: seeking new strategies for self-care of diabetes to share with my health care providers
- Social worker: providing my own emotional support and seeking support for purchasing supplies and coordinating my care
- Hygienist: tending to my skin and my teeth

Some felt that they were activists and advocates.

- Insurance analyst and expert: ready to interpret the health care bill and to negotiate coverage with the insurance company
- Lobbyist: advocating for my needs with my health care provider and employer
- Literary agent: seeking out the best diabetes information and self-help books
- Lawyer: battling for my rights as a woman and a person with diabetes

Are you beginning to see how many hats you wear? Are you surprised at the number of things you are accomplishing? So, what prevents you from consistently fulfilling your responsibilities? Do you tend to put too many things on your "to do" list? Do you include yourself on the list of priorities or do you, like many women, put your needs last? It is time to put yourself at the top of the list. When you are well and happy, your friends and family benefit, too. Congratulate yourself for what you do! Celebrate this awareness with a loved one.

Personality Traits and Job Skills

For any job, people need the right skills and experiences to do the job well. The qualifications for manager of life as a woman with diabetes are quite impressive. If you have or develop these skills, the tasks will be easier to do. Remember, it isn't necessary for you to possess all of these skills. That is why diabetes care involves a partnership between you and your health care provider and between you and your support systems.

Below is a list of unique skills and qualities that you may need both in managing life and in managing diabetes. This list is for your planning and reference. Put a star next to the traits you'd like to develop in the next 6–12 months and a check next to the skills that you already have.

Qualities and Skills

Personality Traits
- ○ Acceptance: loving yourself with all admirable and less than desirable characteristics
- ○ Discipline: following diabetes plan, getting out for the walk, or following the meal plan even when you're not in the mood
- ○ Forgiveness: allowing yourself to make mistakes, to be less than perfect
- ○ Commitment: honoring promises to yourself, following through with intentions despite other requests for your attention

---

Personality Traits (continued)

- ○ Self-reliance: knowing how to help yourself get through the day
- ○ Flexibility: knowing how to go with the flow, to change plans at the last minute, to consider alternative ideas
- ○ Creativity: creating solutions to problems—yours and those of others
- ○ Proficiency: having diabetes self management skills
- ○ Patience: dealing with the unpredictable events in life, the uncooperative blood sugar, and the other people in your life
- ○ Positive self-esteem: knowing that you are worth it; essential when things get tough
- ○ Ingenuity: problem-solving even when the experts are stumped
- ○ Adaptability: meeting unpredictable and crisis situations with flexibility
- ○ Perseverance: never giving up
- ○ Intuition: trusting the inner voice to know when something is not right or when action is needed
- ○ Confidence: feeling capable
- ○ A sense of humor
- ○ Willingness to involve family, friends, partners, and health care providers in aspects of your self-care when you determine what best serves you

Education

- ○ Time management
- ○ Financial management
- ○ Negotiation techniques
- ○ Understanding the causes of high and low blood sugar and how to treat it
- ○ Understanding medical jargon and terminology to decipher physician recommendations, ask questions, and understand the responses

Experience

○ Organizational skills: in health care, home economics, and managing the business operations of your home

○ Communication skills: help others understand your needs and desires (loved ones and health care providers) and clarify goals and intentions for yourself as well

○ Work as part of a team and alone as the situation demands

○ Prioritize demands and solve problems

○ Physical and technical skills: use a glucose meter and lancet device, draw up and inject insulin correctly, record data accurately

○ Analytical and decision-making skills: anticipate the effect of different situations on blood sugar control, make judgments about the best way to correct the problem

○ Health care skills: understand and apply instructions from health care providers to current life issues and long-range health goals

○ Evaluation skills: determine when to reach out for additional support and assistance

Do you have all the skills you need? Do you need some "job training?"

Job Support and Training

The good news is that you are not alone. Many resources are available to help you develop skills and give you the support you need. Diabetes educators can help you improve your diabetes management skills. Local colleges or schools offer a variety of time management, organization, negotiation, and assertiveness courses. Local health clubs, exercise groups, and women's groups, which are often in your local community, can offer you exercise, stress relief, and support.

Growing with the job

Over time you may find that your skills are not enough to reach your current goal or meet the demands on you. Your body will change, resulting in changes in blood sugar levels, medication needs, and overall glycemic control. To meet these evolving demands, you may need to fine-tune your diabetes skills, learn new ones, or develop a different approach to the situation. A diabetes-care provider can help you adjust your treatment program so you can to dine out without experiencing hypoglycemia or help you design a more flexible daily schedule that can change from day to day. You might want to learn more about relaxation techniques to counter the stresses of daily life or time-management strategies to juggle the constant demands of home and work.

Take time to think about how prepared you feel to meet the glycemic goals and life goals you have established for yourself. Begin to think about what new skills you need to achieve these goals. Use the list of personality traits and job skills in the previous section as a guide. Ideas for enhancing your skills and ability to manage life with diabetes will be explored in greater detail in Chapters 4, 5, 6, and 8.

Performance Appraisals and Feedback

Receiving feedback about performance is common in most jobs. For example, a garden grows weeds telling you it needs tending or coworkers compliment you when you've completed an excellent project. With every job, we should receive feedback about our performance. This serves several purposes. Feedback provides us with an opportunity to reflect on our accomplishments. It enables us to develop goals for the future, and to prioritize how we use our time and energy. Performance appraisals also identify what areas need improvement.

Physical feedback

Physical feedback comes in different forms. Test results, such as glycohemoglobin level, your body weight, a cholesterol level, and the glucose checks you do at home, help you evaluate the effectiveness of the care plan or the care choices you make. It is easy to want perfection and to compare yourself to the ideal standard. For instance, you may be tempted to determine your success based on your ability to have the perfect body or HbA$_{1c}$. What standards are you using? Are they realistic? Are they appropriate? Be careful about what standards you use. Check out how realistic they are by discussing them with your health care provider. Remember, these are numbers on the gauges, not the final measure of success. They do not tell the whole story.

Emotional feedback

Performance appraisals also come in the form of verbal feedback from friends and family. Comments like those below can provide you with acknowledgment that what you do counts.

> *I appreciate all that you do.*
> *You manage so many things that other people don't even think*
>   *of ever doing.*
> *Thank you.*

Words of support and encouragement from loved ones can also provide feedback that motivates and keeps you on track.

> *You are working really hard at losing weight.*
> *Keep up the good work. I see you trying.*

Say positive things to yourself whether or not you hear them from others.

The feedback you get from others may not always be what you want to hear. When you are given feedback, first hold it away from you so you can filter it, take it apart, and evaluate what it is worth. Is there some truth in it? If there is, explore how you can use it. If not, then let it go. Constructive feedback, even though it is painful, can be helpful to focus your attention on developing a healthier approach to achieving wellness. It is important for you to learn how to filter the feedback you get and decide whether it is worth considering or discarding.

Spiritual feedback

The most important performance appraisal comes from honestly reflecting on yourself. Details on skills and tools to help you evaluate yourself and to develop an action plan are in Chapter 5.

The Working Environment

Diabetes consists of a 168-hour, 7-day work week with no vacations or weekends! The schedule you keep for glycemic control may not coincide with the schedule your family keeps or with your other work and social life. You are expected to work with your diabetes in an environment that can be unpredictable.

Examine the nature of your environment—the physical demands, the emotional challenges, the support systems. Identify what is chaotic and stressful, what is productive and supportive. Think about who is there to listen and to help you in your quest for health and wellness? Be gentle as you begin to unveil the elements of your world. Be honest about what or who depletes your energy. Notice what or who recharges and supports you. If the demands seem too great or the environment is harsh, consider reaching out for the support and guidance needed to protect and nourish you. This is your right. Here are some hints for coping.

1. Give yourself a pat on the back! You do a lot!
2. Work with someone to figure out how you can change your diabetes schedule to coordinate it with your daily tasks.
3. Do not give up, even when you have unexpected highs and lows! Know that things outside of your control sometimes affect your blood sugar level.

You may occasionally be surrounded by a well intentioned chorus telling you what to do and how to do it. Or uninvited advisors telling you what you should or shouldn't do, criticizing you for the choices you make. Try to remain calm. Even your health care providers may not understand why your glucose targets have eluded you. Here are some hints for coping.

1. Be honest with yourself about what you are doing, and decide whether you are acting in your best interest.
2. Remember that you have the right to make choices, even when others don't agree. You also have the right not to share all the reasons why you do what you do.
3. Be careful not to take what is said personally. Tell your ego to be quiet. Take in all the suggestions, keep the ones you find valuable, and discard the rest.
4. Take a deep breath. Consider thanking the choir and telling them that you will let them know when you need support.
5. Remember, you don't have to be perfect.

Benefits

How often do you stop to appreciate the experiences you have every day? The fast pace of today's world easily draws us into overdrive and fatigue. We are trying to overcome even the natural limitations of time and energy. We fill our lives with enough for a 40-hour day! How often do you *stop* to take a deep breath; "stop to smell the flowers?"

Taking a coffee break or a day off is part of the work culture. Most people who work have some time off, a weekend, a vacation, or even sick time. The purpose of this time off is to rest and recharge for the work week ahead. Without this time, employees burn out, are less productive, and have more sick days.

A critical but often unexplored aspect of your career with diabetes is creating this essential benefit, time to recharge and replenish your energy. Energy is stored in physical, emotional, and spiritual banks. You draw on these energy accounts to deal with the daily tasks that include diabetes. These are also the stores that help you through those crises with diabetes. It takes a great deal of energy to deal with a crisis. When your resources are limited or depleted, you can't cope well. It is easy to misinterpret events and react out of hurt or fatigue instead of responding to the actual event.

Have you ever considered taking a vacation from diabetes or from your day-to-day responsibilities? Creating vacation time is being good to yourself. Relaxation and rest allow you the space to listen to your body, spirit, and emotions. Now is the time to explore how to do this and protect your greatest investment—yourself. Okay, you can't park the diabetes on a shelf and come back Monday to pick it up. But you could unload some of your responsibilities. You could ask a loved one or a diabetes provider to review the blood sugar measurements and determine changes in insulin dose. Or you might negotiate with someone else to do the cooking, cleaning, or shopping for a few days. Taking a day off or a vacation will mean different things to different people. What will give you a rest and time to get reacquainted with yourself?

Take time out! Explore how you can
with a friend or a loved one. You are worth it!

My Vacation or "Time Off" Will Be...

Transitions

Consider again your diabetes job responsibilities with greater appreciation for the day-to-day tasks that achieve wellness. This career is a challenge! The demands are high. When you realize all the demands on your time and energy, you can appreciate why it is so important to nurture and take care of yourself.

This is the time to take stock and commit to yourself. Direct some of your caring energy inward. Make yourself a priority. The key is to listen, learn, and respond to the wisdom of your own body. Managing life as a woman with diabetes provides you with a powerful opportunity to discover more about your own wonderful qualities and to express yourself in new ways. Take a moment now to give yourself a pat on the back, a hug, and words of appreciation. You are a remarkable woman.

Self-Assessment

This checklist outlines the responsibilities of women who manage life and diabetes. With a friend or by yourself, identify which responsibilities are yours alone and which ones you can share with another person. Put a check next to those duties you already do well. Place a star next to those you feel are important and worth doing better.

Responsibilities of Manager of Diabetes

Do well	Need to do	General Self-Care
○	○	Rest when you need to. If you are tired, stop and give your body a break. Practice relaxation techniques.
○	○	Get plenty of sleep.
○	○	Exercise regularly.
○	○	Drink 6–8 cups of caffeine-free, alcohol-free, sugar-free fluids each day.
○	○	Lubricate your skin if it is dry.
○	○	Seek out emotional assistance if life is overwhelming and if you are feeling sad.
○	○	Determine what your needs are and seek ways to meet them.
○	○	Prioritize your needs and the needs of others. Determine how to balance them. Share the tasks.

Do well	Need to do	**General Self-Care (continued)**
◯	◯	Respect your body and the unique health need that it has.
◯	◯	Accept other people's help.
◯	◯	Engage in activities that allow you to be creative; do things you enjoy.

Home Care (May or may not be shared with a spouse or roommate.)

◯	◯	Do the shopping and cooking.
◯	◯	Do the cleaning and laundry.
◯	◯	Do maintenance and home repair.
◯	◯	Keep the lawn mowed, the garden tended.
◯	◯	Empty the garbage routinely.

Other People Care

Child care

◯	◯	Feed and clothe the children.
◯	◯	Keep watch and respond to their ongoing developmental and health care needs.
◯	◯	Comfort them when sad or scared. Celebrate their joys.
◯	◯	Bathe them and tuck them in.
◯	◯	Get them off to school or day care on time and safely.
◯	◯	Help them off to college or transition into adult hood.
◯	◯	Organize social outings, all the way from preparing to cleaning up and putting away.
◯	◯	Function as the diplomat and mediator in the family, seeking to keep peace between all family members and resolve the small wars that seem to present themselves.

Do well	Need to do	Other People Care (continued)
○	○	Serve as the confidant, advisor, and informer, always prepared to have your ideas discarded or argued with.
○	○	Baby-sit and care for grandchildren when and if the opportunity presents itself.

Parent care

Do well	Need to do	
○	○	Bring parent to doctor appointments and help address the effects of current illnesses.
○	○	Develop strategies to ensure safety and comfort.
○	○	Do the cooking, cleaning, and home repairs as needed.
○	○	Assist with financial management and personal care as needed.
○	○	Share creative activities.

Relationships

Do well	Need to do	
○	○	Respond to the needs and desires of your spouse or partner.
○	○	Communicate your needs and desires calmly and clearly.
○	○	Negotiate conflicts smoothly.
○	○	Give time to the relationship even when it means delaying going to bed at the end of an exhausting day.
○	○	Do something special for that extra special somebody in your life.
○	○	Receive gifts, suggestions, and even criticism gracefully. Figure out what is important to you so you can learn more about yourself.
○	○	Cook and entertain.

Do well	Need to do	**Other People Care (continued)**
○	○	Be open to asking for support and letting others support your efforts.
○	○	Work well as a team.

Diabetes Self-Care

Do well	Need to do	
○	○	Choose what and when to eat.
○	○	Monitor your blood sugar as often as you and your health care provider decide is best.
○	○	Enjoy some physical activity every day.
○	○	Respond to blood sugar levels that are outside of desired range.
○	○	Check your feet daily, washing and lubricating them as needed.
○	○	Take your medications in the right amount, at the right time, and using the right technique.
○	○	If you take insulin, adjust the dose after careful consideration of the factors that can cause your blood sugar to go too high or low.
○	○	See a dietitian or nurse educator at least once a year.
○	○	See your doctor routinely, 2–4 times a year.
○	○	Together with your providers determine goals for diabetes. Work out the small steps it will take to reach your goal.
○	○	Apply the diabetes care principles that you learn.
○	○	Watch to see how your choices and behaviors affect glucose control and overall health.
○	○	Tell your provider what parts of the plan are difficult or not working for you.
○	○	Determine what your needs are and communicate them. Ask for help when you are tired or unable to pay attention to your needs.

Do well	Need to do	**Diabetes Self-Care (continued)**
○	○	Think through the steps you need to take to prevent and to treat high and low blood sugar.
○	○	Work as captain of the team.

Risk Factor Reduction

Do well	Need to do	
○	○	If you smoke, stop. Or look into smoking cessation programs.
○	○	If you have high blood pressure, cholesterol or triglycerides, follow a meal plan and take prescribed medications to bring levels into the desired range.
○	○	If you are overweight, alter your eating and activity habits.

Employment (for those who also work outside the home)

Do well	Need to do	
○	○	Complete projects and responsibilities as requested.
○	○	Maintain professionalism at all times.
○	○	Conduct yourself in a customer-friendly manner.
○	○	Do not let home and social life interfere with work.
○	○	Be efficient and courteous.
○	○	Accommodate the job assignments from your employer while simultaneously taking care of the household and family.

There are many job responsibilities. You do not have to do them all by yourself. Sharing them with others will help you achieve wellness and live a full and balanced life.

Chapter 3

Moving Along Your Own Career Path

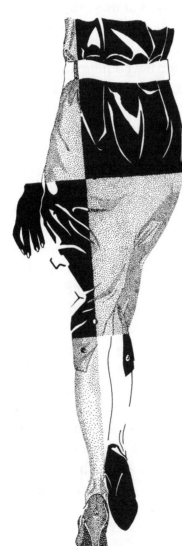

*Travel not only stirs
the blood. It also gives
strength to the spirit.*
    —Florance Prag Kahn

As a woman with diabetes, you travel three intertwined pathways as you move through your life.

1. Diabetes: the pathway of diabetes acceptance, from diagnosis and denial to accepting diabetes as part of you.
2. Life: the pathway of development through life's stages, from birth through adulthood and ending in death.
3. Wellness: the pathway of health awareness, from treating and feeling better about illness and disability to enhancing personal health and well-being to reach full potential.

Your own career path is composed of these three pathways. One (Diabetes) is the stages of acceptance that you go through in learning to live with any chronic disease (from denying you have it to accepting it as part of who you are). Another pathway (Life) is the stages of life that you move through as you develop, take on new responsibilities, and meet the associated challenges. The third pathway (Wellness) involves increasing self awareness, which leads to personal health and well-being. These pathways braid together to form your career path. If you undo this braid and think carefully about each strand, you won't get them tangled up! This will give you insight into how to invest your time and energy into yourself.

You do not travel these pathways one at a time, nor without retracing steps, taking detours, and hitting impasses. Smooth travel on one path fosters smoother travel on another. Sometimes the paths merge and managing your "career" (diabetes, life, and health) seems effortless. At other times nothing is easy. You may find yourself struggling to find the way as the demands of your life, diabetes, and health clash. Understanding where you are on each pathway will give you insight into what matters at that place. Then you can make plans for your health and happiness. As you would on any career path, you progress as you learn, experience, and become motivated to take on new challenges.

First, let's discover where you are on each pathway and learn how that place influences your choices. Second, let's braid the three pathways together to see how they shape your response to your life as a woman with diabetes. We hope that along the way you will identify a few things in your life worth paying special attention to and develop some strategies for setting and reaching your self-care goals.

The Pathway of Diabetes Acceptance

Accepting diabetes happens gradually and is a continual process. Acceptance is not being problem-free, but accepting the problems as just another part of who you are. The pathway of diabetes acceptance is cyclical in nature. As you come to terms with one aspect of having diabetes, you are ready to deal with another aspect and the acceptance process begins again. After learning how to follow a meal plan based on exchanges and accepting eyeballing or measuring portion sizes as part of your eating habit, you may become frustrated when you begin a serious diet and want to match what you eat with your exercise and medication. Carbohydrate counting appears to be the answer, but the idea of reading labels again makes you hesitate before starting the new meal plan. You need to go through the process of acceptance for this diet change just as you did when you adopted your original meal plan.

There are two different aspects of acceptance here. First, you accept diabetes as part of who you are. Second, you accept what you need to do to live with it. Time and life events affect your motivation, resources, and need to take care of yourself. How you relate to yourself as a woman with diabetes is unique. You are the only one who understands what having diabetes is really like for you. However, the process of accepting diabetes does follow predictable steps.

Look at the levels of diabetes acceptance listed on the next page. Identify where you are now.

Levels of Diabetes Acceptance

1. Moving in

This initial step begins with diagnosis and involves "learning the ropes." Through experimenting and learning, you will determine how to adopt the new responsibilities delegated to you. You begin to realize what strengths, resources, and influence you can bring to the new challenge. Feelings of shock, fear, and anger are common. You can return to this level as you experience changes in your life, health, and diabetes care. For example, at first you exercise at 6 a.m. every day for 30 minutes in order to avoid hypoglycemia. You may wish to change to exercising at other times of the day as you begin to understand how exercise affects your blood sugar levels and learn that a glass of juice before exercising usually prevents hypoglycemia.

2. Moving through

This more settled phase happens as you develop regular diabetes care habits and learn how to cope with unplanned events. You reach a plateau, a level of comfort and familiarity. You may feel more confident. Many people become bored with the routine and frustrated by the unpredictability associated with diabetes. The new demand—to maintain your commitment and interest—is far greater than the demands during the first stage when it was new and promising.

3. Moving along

This phase of renewal involves more change. It occurs when you realize that your approach no longer matches your current situation and needs. It is from the work done in his phase that you identify new goals and expectations. You begin to see yourself in a new way. The challenge here is to *take stock* of where you are and to *take charge* of getting to where you want to be.

Moving in

With no prior experience and little preparation, you are suddenly awarded a new position in life. And you must begin training promptly because it will become a full-blown career. Things move very quickly on diagnosis (the hiring process). Often, the new hire is trained to be a walking encyclopedia of diabetes facts, without anyone ever considering how to fit the care plan (job expectations) with your past "job experience" and competing demands for your money, time, and energy.

You need diabetes training to occur gradually over time because absorbing new information and integrating changes in your lifestyle takes time. You may feel overwhelmed and at the mercy of the health care team members who are telling you what to do. You'll probably go through some form of denial at this stage. It's normal whenever you have to adjust to an unexpected event. All of us resist change and cling to our familiar lifestyle, even if it doesn't work for us anymore.

Try to learn about diabetes in manageable chunks. At first you just need to know what to do each day to survive. It is very important to share the details about your everyday lifestyle and schedule with the health care team so you can work together to develop a diabetes care plan that fits. If it doesn't fit you, you won't wear it. You are the only one who knows what will work for you. This is an important job responsibility. After "moving in" you are in line to be promoted to the head of your health care team. Your health care team is actually working for you to fit the new demands of diabetes in with the rest of your life.

Moving through

After recovering from the initial shock of being told you had diabetes, you begin to form beliefs about why you developed it, who you are now, and what you will need to do differently. For example, many people think that eating too much sugar causes diabetes (but it doesn't). Many people believe that you can't ever eat sugar again if you have diabetes (but you can). These beliefs may be at the heart of your refusal to follow your meal plan now. You need to look at what you believe about diabetes to see if those beliefs are limiting your growth. The information, support, and guidance you received at diagnosis helped shape your current beliefs, but you should evaluate them now and replace those that no longer serve you well.

Moving along

You may not always be thinking about your diabetes and for the most part, you feel like you accept it. Then, without warning, something happens (developing retinopathy, having a serious insulin reaction, being rejected by the man you love), that challenges this level of acceptance. Once again, you need to spend time getting comfortable with your diabetes in order to move along.

It is hard to accept such a complicated challenge, especially when you didn't ask for or expect it. Yet, unless you reach a sense of wholeness as a woman who happens to have diabetes, your energy gets locked up in fighting or denying it, preventing you from fulfilling other needs.

What is the most difficult part of having diabetes for you right now? How did you resolve earlier challenges? What about having diabetes do you ignore? How has your attitude to having diabetes changed since the first year after being diagnosed?

Let's look at how two different women "moved in" with diabetes and are continuing to "move through" it.

Hanna, now 37, was 5 years old when she was diagnosed with diabetes. She vividly remembers this and how she decided that having diabetes wasn't going to change her life.

> *She remembers being in the hospital. She was overjoyed with all the attention she was getting. She even enjoyed being in a cage-bed full of toys and being able to ask the nurse for juice whenever she wanted. Grape juice parties with the little boy in the next bed were fun. Hanna would reach through the bars and say "cheers" before gulping down her juice. She couldn't understand why her parents seemed so concerned. She understood that things were not OK when the nurse answered her request*

for another juice party with "Hanna, you can't have grape juice anymore. You have diabetes." This was the first of many painful realizations and changes. But she was determined not to let anything wreck her parties. She replaced juice parties with swapping toys with the little boy. Taking shots and weighing food were like brushing her teeth. She quickly learned that if she did what "they" asked her to, she could do most of what she wanted to. This is still the way Hanna views having diabetes. She keeps herself relatively in control and leads her life as she pleases. She'll find a way to see the positive even when things are really bad. Hanna remarked, "Looking back, I think that because I have diabetes, I look harder for things to celebrate, take greater risks, and work harder to accomplish more than most people."

Dorothy, now 58, was diagnosed when she was 47. Her diagnosis was a blur. She hardly remembers when she first began to feel bad but remembers clearly realizing how much her daily routine would be forever changed by the diagnosis. She first became aware that something was wrong when she was on vacation, visiting her sister.

She felt groggy and sick to her stomach. Her sister asked her if she was depressed or sick. She was not having much fun on the vacation she needed so badly but felt OK. On her sister's recommendation, she called her doctor when she got home. The next day, after a long morning of tests, she learned that she had diabetes. She was shocked. She knew something was wrong but never imagined that she was that sick. She knew nothing about diabetes and was terrified. Dorothy had lost her job six months before. She was sure her diabetes was a result of the stress. She had already asked friends and family for support, now what was she going to do? She couldn't imagine how she was going to afford all the supplies that she needed. She asked, "Why me" and "Why now?" Developing diabetes at a time when so much else was going on and money was tight made accepting it more of a challenge. Dorothy felt burdened and still feels angry about the demands that having diabetes places on her. "At one time, I stopped taking my medication. I convinced myself that I didn't really need the pills, but really I just hated spending the money on them."

It took her 11 years, most of them in denial, but she can say that now she is facing her diabetes, things are much better. She thought she had freedom when she was eating what she wanted to and not thinking about diabetes at all, but it wasn't freedom. It was jail. She felt angry all the time and was too tired to go out. She had to convince herself that giving up eating fried chicken everyday wasn't going to deprive her of her freedom. She had to realize that taking care of herself was a good thing. "I still feel angry at times, but mostly I get mad at myself for not doing what I need to do."

It is important to connect with your own diagnosis story. It is always an emotional event in a woman's life. When you take on the job of diabetes, you are very vulnerable to the suggestions and attitudes of those around you. You may have felt powerful negative emotions at the reactions and attitudes of the health care professionals and your family and friends. You need to recognize how you felt then because these emotions may still be coloring your viewpoint and responses now.

To move through the levels of acceptance, you need to know what level you are on, what issues you don't accept, and what challenges diabetes brings you. From here you will be able to develop a more concrete plan moving you toward wellness.

The Pathway of Life

Life takes us through predictable stages. During each stage, you are presented with challenges, and you gain knowledge and grow

Diabetes Diagnosis Exercise

How old were you when you developed diabetes?

_____

What responsibilities did you have and how confident in meeting them were you?

_____

What financial challenges were you faced with?

_____

What was your first reaction to the definitive diagnosis of diabetes?

_____

What initial reaction and expression of support did close family and friends provide?

_____

What was your relationship like with your health care providers?

_____

Did you understand what was happening to your body and why?

_____

Were there people available to answer your questions and help you integrate the demands of diabetes into your life?

_____

Were your initial needs taken care of?

_____

What lingering needs from your initial diagnosis are still unmet?

_____

by meeting those challenges. What you learn in each stage enables you to grow into the next stage. You may need to retrace your steps as you develop and find new ways to move through old issues. The experiences you have shape who you are. First, look at the life stages listed below and the issues that often come with them.

Life Stages

Getting out on your own
- developing confidence in peers, co-workers, superiors, and community
- conforming to friends
- developing an intimate committed partnership
- deciding about marriage
- selecting and preparing for an occupation
- starting a new job
- feeling lonely
- experiencing pregnancy and childbirth
- leaving home
- experimenting with family values
- achieving independence from parents (emotional, & financial)

Discovering who you are
- searching for identity
- developing/nurturing partnership
- considering/starting a family
- dreaming about your future

- taking on major responsibilities
- developing satisfying social groups
- working toward personal goals
- deepening friendships
- asking "who am I?"
- doing what you "should"
- making commitments
- beginning/nurturing a career

Raising questions
- having/raising children
- settling down
- advancing in your career
- accommodating to multiple-roles
- asking "what do I want to do with my life?"
- desiring freedom
- declining satisfaction in marriage/ partnership
- divorce
- recognizing personal limitations

Changing perspectives

- learning to play again
- experiencing peak competency
- emotional turmoil
- accommodating to limits of personal power
- changing careers
- moving
- asking "what about me?"
- changing physical activity
- parenting teenagers
- asking deep questions
- remarriage
- having a sense of aloneness
- awareness of mortality
- death of a person close to you

Enjoying more freedom

- experiencing menopause
- beginning to consider/plan for retirement
- acting on new values
- adjusting to empty nest
- selecting a few good friends
- adjusting to grandparenting
- Reviewing personal, relationship, and career goals
- supporting aging parents
- enjoying life
- enjoying more financial freedom

Deepening sense of purpose

- softening feelings
- adjusting to limitations
- dealing with financial pressures
- quiet joys
- facing death
- death of loved one/close friend
- making new friends
- loss of energy
- retirement
- developing steady commitments to self and others

Entering the twilight

- experiencing loneliness
- depending on those who once depended on you
- seeking companionship
- having trouble with memory
- sense of peace and perspective
- freedom from "shoulds"
- losing partner and friends
- preparing for death
- difficulty getting around
- experiencing physical challenges
- enjoying the present moment

—*adapted from* Kicking Your Stress Habits, *Donald Tubesing, 1989.*

Each phase has its own unique qualities and impact on a woman. Let's take a moment to identify where you are and which situations you have already experienced.

What Stage Are You In Now?

1. Find which stage matches your life right now. Which issues listed below this stage have you experienced?

2. Look at earlier stages. Put a check next to the issues you have already dealt with.

3. Pat yourself on the back for all of your effort and growing as you moved through these situations.

4. Circle all the issues you are working with now. Keep these in mind as you work through the book and decide where and how to use your energy for self-care.

Now, in the exercise on the next page, identify your current stage in life and the challenges you are facing.

Life change

At each stage in your life, you must adapt to changes. What you learn from changing and what you do to handle the associated stress (your coping style) defines who you are.

Change always challenges us, but each new challenge is an opportunity. Facing challenges (and opportunities) can be stressful. For example, you left your family as a young adult and set up your own household. Leaving home challenged you to set up and keep house and to organize your finances. This is part of growing up. Above all else, and no matter what, you can expect change. It's normal and inevitable. Demands on your time will come and go.

Life Stage Exercise

What general life stage are you in right now?

_____

_____

What are the major challenges of this life stage for you?

_____

_____

_____

Did you struggle with certain issues in earlier stages that you are feeling more confident about handling now?

_____

_____

_____

What one skill (time management, budgeting, communication, negotiation, stress management, etc.), if you had it mastered, would help you the most in dealing with your life challenges now?

_____

_____

Responsibilities shift. Self-image evolves. Friendships wane. Energy fluctuates. Bodies grow and change.

As a woman with a chronic illness, you can expect to be challenged financially, physically, and emotionally. Meeting these challenges can seem overwhelming at times. It will help you to remember that being challenged pushes you to draw on your own wit and wisdom to develop new skills and strategies. You have the opportunity to discover that you can do more than you thought. You can bloom and grow in your job. And these skills are transferable! For example, bearing the constant financial burdens of diabetes may have forced you to budget more carefully, create a rainy-day bank account, and check your insurance claims to be sure they were being properly handled. When you retire, these habits will serve you well as you navigate the maze of Medicare and enjoy the money you put away. This is just one example of the training that makes every woman with diabetes better equipped to deal with the expected challenges of living.

As human beings, as women, and as individuals with diabetes, we move through stages of life and come to new levels of understanding. Your age, stage in life, responsibilities, coping style, and resources play a big part in how you respond to change and how quickly you can accept and fit diabetes into your life.

The Pathway of Wellness

As we said in Chapter 1, you can have physical health problems and still feel well. Wellness is wholeness—a blend of body, mind, and soul. Wellness is about consistently making choices that enhance, rather than jeopardize, your health and well-being. It is now commonly accepted that if you approach life positively and do things regularly to promote your well-being, you can affect how well and even how long you live.

You are not simply focused on what's wrong with you and getting relief, but on what's right and living to the fullest! Wellness is not simply the absence of illness or injury. Its an attitude and a way of approaching your life. Your personal wellness depends on being tuned-in to yourself and seeking care and knowledge in order to thrive. Your regular routines, what you think, and how you react to things are the guideposts along this path. You will need to examine how you react to stress (adversity) and how your reactions influence your physical and mental well-being. Do you take a hot bath at the end of an exhausting day, feeling proud of all you accomplished as you relax tense muscles and foster a good nights sleep? Or, feeling depleted, do you drink a few glasses of wine to unwind, fostering hypoglycemia at 2 a.m. and a sleepless night? Let's look at how you navigate along this path. Psychologist Albert

Ellis explained the ABCs of behavior in *How to Stubbornly Refuse to Make Yourself Miserable About Anything, Yes, Anything!*

Adversity—anything that causes you to react.

Beliefs—what you think and how you feel about the adversity.

Consequences—your reaction to your *beliefs* about the adversity.

The ABCs may give you a new key to understanding how you developed your routines, got into the ruts, or nourished the resiliency you experience today. By understanding where behavior begins, you can take steps to get out of the ruts and develop more healthful routines. This means making changes and consciously paying attention to things happening around you. Moving toward wellness involves looking out for yourself and balancing the various aspects of your health. Below are the steps to this process. You will spiral upward through these steps on your way along the wellness path.

Making Healthful Changes

Realize—What belief or behavior do I want to change to enhance my health and well-being?

Vitalize—Determine something you can *do* to make this change.

Prioritize—Decide how you want to make it happen. Find the necessary time, approval, money, space, or motivation you need. Figure out how you will deal with any barriers that may get in your way.

Synthesize—Practice it, refine it, and make it part of you. Incorporate the new belief or behavior into your regular routine and *self-concept.*

Revitalize—As this belief or practice becomes out-of-date with your realities, begin the cycle again.

Diagram of Healthful Change

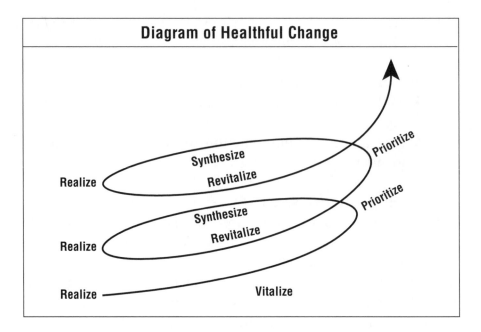

Self-care Exercise

What was the most recent belief or behavior you changed in caring for yourself as a person with diabetes (for example, starting an exercise program)?

_____

_____

1. Realize
How did you become aware that you wanted/needed to do this? Where did you get help in learning various ways to do it?

_____

_____

2. Vitalize
How did you decide what to do? Did you list many different ways?

_____

_____

Which one did you choose?

_____

_____

3. Prioritize

List anything that you felt would make it difficult to adopt the new behavior or belief. How did you deal with these barriers?

_____

_____

What did you have to overcome or make happen to adopt the new behavior or belief?

_____

_____

4. Synthesize

Describe the process of fitting this new practice into your lifestyle and dealing with the barriers you listed above.

_____

_____

What did you learn about yourself in this process?

_____

_____

5. Revitalize

What changes have you needed to make to this belief or behavior over time?

_____

_____

_____

Can you see any life changes in the future that might require you to revitalize your current practice?

The career path: life, diabetes, and wellness

We all move through predictable phases when we change. Whether the change was planned, like deciding to wear an insulin pump, or unexpected, like being suddenly diagnosed with diabetes, these same phases occur. For women the most profound changes usually occur during adolescence, the consummation of a relationship, the birth of a child, the death of a loved one, a move, a job change, any change in family composition, a serious health problem, or menopause. The way you responded to any of these events reveals your coping style. If you are not satisfied with it, get support and adopt a new one that works better for you.

Any job has predictable phases, too. Learn the ropes, acquire new skills, become competent, reach goals, and after some time at the same job, watch for burnout. You will go through each one of these phases. In fact, you probably have gone through them over the years in caring for yourself, raising children, volunteering, managing a household, or working as an employee. You may have already learned that you have to revitalize yourself to get out of the burnout stage. You need to take time to evaluate where you are and where you want to go. Then you find the inspiration—perhaps from a friend, a book, or a class—to head off in a new direction. This is the process that helps you change. This is how you enrich your experiences—and get better results on the job.

Chapter 4

Support: Communicating on the Job

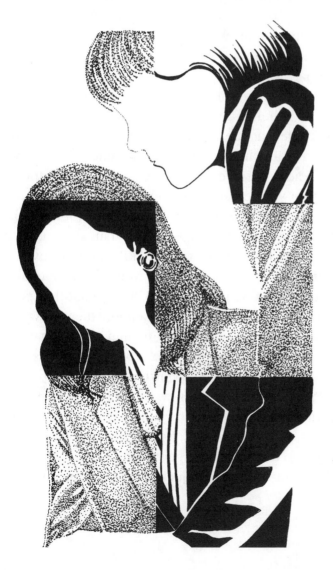

I believe the greatest gift I can conceive of having from anyone is to be seen by them, heard by them, to be understood and touched by them. The greatest gift I can give is to see, hear, understand, and to touch another person. When this is done, I feel contact has been made.
—Virginia Satir

Learning to communicate effectively is a central life skill for every one. It will give you an edge in building strong relationships and handling the difficult ones. It will help you to work with doctors to determine which treatment will fit your needs the best. The motivation to polish up communication and negotiation skills comes from wanting the best life has to offer and wanting to give your best to the people you love.

Wanting to be there for the people you love is one of the most powerful motivations for taking care of yourself. As you age, grow, and develop, you redefine what being there means. But it always involves listening and connecting with the people in your life. The truth is that being there for yourself is the key to being *able* to be there for others. In this chapter we explore what being supported and being supportive is all about. We examine how you can build more meaningful relationships.

Developing meaningful relationships may be the single best way to promote your well-being and prolong your life. Having relationships with people who are supportive is basic to your health. Maintaining these relationships requires confidence, trust, and interpersonal skills. The skill and confidence to deal with the strains that diabetes places on your existing relationships takes practice. How, then, do you acquire the necessary skills? It is not realistic to expect to get this training in a routine doctor visit, so you need to take the responsibility for acquiring these skills on your own.

It can be very lonely living with diabetes. Mutually-supportive relationships help dissolve this loneliness. Allowing another person to support you opens a door for you to support them in ways they may otherwise never experience. Giving and receiving support builds trust between two people. This trust strengthens the relationship. Your ability to create and nurture relationships will be tested as you move in and out of new situations. When you decide to confide in another person, how s/he perceives diabetes may determine how s/he relates to you. Some people may choose to shy away from you out of fear and ignorance. Worse, you may shy away from them out of fear of rejection or being misunderstood.

In Chapter 1, we looked at how women view having diabetes. You need to look closely at what having diabetes really means to you and how it changes the way you relate to others. Checking another person's understanding of diabetes and providing them with more accurate information can clear up a lot. Modern medical and nutritional advances have liberated you to lead a more independent life. People who are not familiar with diabetes don't know about these advances. The average person's perception of life with diabetes often comes from their memories of grandma at a time when diabetes meant restrictions and a bleak outlook. This is not true today with blood glucose monitoring, variety of medication options, and new medical tests to identify complications early and ways to treat them. To separate fact from fiction, stay current with diabetes developments and share these with others.

Putting the knowledge and technology into practice is liberating, but it is also demanding of your time and energy and often is expensive. Further, deciding among all the options available to you creates an additional burden and strain on relationships. It is easy to make your diabetes the culprit for failed relationships, even when having it has nothing to do with the problem. Developing and living with diabetes, like anything that is stressful, magnifies any existing problem in a relationship.

Your Support Network

People can support, be indifferent to, or interfere with your efforts to care for yourself. In any successful interaction, information is communicated, emotions are expressed, and agreements are reached. It is your responsibility to get your point across, to handle your emotions, and to make agreements that work for you. Which people in your life support you? Who interferes? How easily do you relate to them?

In the box on the next page, list the people or groups of people in your life now. Include partners, children, relatives, friends, work and volunteer associates, and other people who are important to you.

List of the Support People in Your Life

Intimate partner _____

Children _____

Friends _____

Family _____

Work and/or volunteer associates _____

Health care providers _____

Others _____

Go back to your list. Circle those who generally support you and underline those who don't.

What are your reactions to your list? List those emotions in the space below. Acknowledge these and think about how you would like to feel about each person on your list.

_____
_____
_____
_____

Your feelings about people who are there for you and about those who are not can color your own view of having diabetes and affect how you handle it. You cannot change another person. But you can change yourself. Work on your own interpersonal skills and try to negotiate a new way of relating to each other. There isn't one right way to assist another person. Each person that you listed above has a unique relationship with you, understanding of what you need, and style of helping you.

Susan still vividly remembers a stranger she counts among the most supportive people she has ever known. Just released from the hospital, hungry and exhausted from her recent surgery, she attempted to maneuver the cafeteria line with her luggage. As her blood sugar dropped rapidly, she was overwhelmed by the task of buying lunch. The attendant saw her need, called another attendant to cover the register, picked up Susan's tray, and escorted her to a nearby table. She placed Susan's tray on the table, put her luggage on a nearby chair, and said, "Have a good lunch."

Someone really cared and helped Susan in a time of need. Almost nothing was said between the two women, but the warm compassion expressed by a stranger will always remind Susan that people do care. Support comes in different ways. Look at the ways you are supported.

Now think of the people you turn to for the types of support listed on the next page. Write their names next to the roles they play in your life.

How do you define being *supportive?* How do "they" define being supportive? Everyone reacts differently to another person's attempts to listen, understand, and help them. What feels supportive for one person can be irritating for another. Letting others know what is supportive to you makes it easier and more rewarding for them to help.

Helping other people help you

It is natural to reject people's efforts to help when they are not useful, or are even irritating. Again, clear communication helps others know what you really need from them, even if it is nothing. It is your responsibility to tell other people what you need. It is especially important to tell them when they have really supported you. This strengthens your relationship and allows them to enjoy the feeling of being there.

If you look from their point of view, you may realize that trying to help you, especially if you are ambivalent about doing what you

Who Do You Turn To?

For cheerleading _____

For help with personal problems _____

For direction and clarification _____

For expert diabetes advice _____

To share problems _____

For respect and approval _____

For energy and motivation _____

To provide for you (financial, housing, food, etc.) _____

_____

_____

For inspiration _____

For an honest opinion _____

Do you feel supported by the people you listed above?

_____

_____

Who do you shut out when he or she tries to help?

_____

Who offers support in a way that you really appreciate?

_____

_____

need to do, is tricky. It isn't easy to offer support that is rejected. It can be frustrating and irritating for them. It is difficult to watch someone you love struggle doing something that seems fairly simple to you.

Roberta dreaded the day she saw coming when her pills would be replaced by insulin shots. She swore to herself and her husband, Harry, that she would never give herself a shot. Her anger and stubbornness bothered Harry. How could this woman who raised four children and balanced the finances for his business for 35 years refuse to do what the doctor said? He joked with her about it, but his jokes made her even angrier.

Harry thought this task would be easy. He didn't realize that the idea of giving shots was very intimidating to his wife. This simple technical skill was associated with fear and painful memories for her. Roberta needed to share these memories with Harry. As a small child, she watched her Aunt Harriet give herself shots in the kitchen before meals. Diabetes took Harriet's life, after it took one leg and made her almost blind. After Roberta explained to Harry, he understood that she wasn't ready to face giving her own injections. She didn't want to end up like Harriet. Then Harry could be compassionate and help her put things in perspective. Going on insulin will probably help her get better control of her blood sugars, and better control can stop or slow down those scary complications.

Often women (and people with diabetes) refuse to ask for help. Fearing rejection or being put down is common. Needing to appear to be in control often gets in the way of asking for the assistance you need while you are learning to cope. Having your feelings misread is common. You may not be aware of how you are expressing yourself. Your emotional reactions can be hard even for you to understand. Giving yourself ample time to adjust and turning to other people for help while you adapt to diabetes is a sign of inner strength.

Part of being in a loving relationship is being clear in your communication. Loving other people doesn't mean they can read your mind. Being aware of yourself is the first step to good communication. This can be difficult when you are in the thick of accepting change. Change is messy and uncomfortable. The people who know you well can help if you let them. Another person's more objective perspective may help you gain valuable insight.

Strengthened by other people's nurturing and respect, you can adapt more easily and securely to change. Your part in assisting them to support you is as important as their part. Realize what you are asking of the people who want to support you. Here are some examples of support commonly desired by women with diabetes. Each is followed by a phrase illustrating how the need could be communicated.

- Be understanding and patient. "It's not easy to balance all my responsibilities."
- Be accepting of me. "Sometimes I just need time to absorb it all."
- Be positive and upbeat. "Help me keep my sense of humor."
- Applaud what I am doing. "I need to realize that I am working hard, even if my glucose meter reads 200!"
- Be supportive. "I need to know you believe in me."
- Be involved. "I need your help in figuring it all out."
- Just be there for me. "I know that I am the one who has diabetes, but knowing you are there makes a real difference."

Social Skills for Health and Wellness

Checking your blood sugar is concrete. You do it, and it is done. Relating to people when you are experiencing highs and lows is the real work. Preparing healthy meals is easy compared to relating to a child or spouse who refuses to eat them. The people you relate to—your social network—and the way you relate to them define your social life. Those people who are there for you no matter what are as valuable as your glucose meter. Clear communication and negotiation are vital skills for good relations with other people. This work has three parts: clarify what you want to communicate, get the message across, and make agreements to get what you, or they, need.

Clarify what you want to communicate

Communication is a two way street. The better you are at being clear, the easier it will be to get your message across. Take the time to straighten out your thoughts, think about how you want your message to be heard, and reflect on the best time to communicate before you utter a word. This will boost your success at getting your message across. There are a few other elements to consider.

Deciding whether or not to share information. Not sharing information is a valid choice. You have the right to choose what you will share and when. But, relationships are based on two people sharing experiences, thoughts, ideas, and dreams. Sharing things that you have difficulty thinking about takes courage. A woman who chose not to tell a close friend that she had diabetes might be considered rude when she declined a piece of surprise birthday cake. Her choice not to tell makes her responsible for the strain on the relationship. A good way to determine what you need to share and when is to ask yourself, "Does her/his knowing that I have diabetes matter to me or our relationship?"

Being truthful. It is hard to admit that you haven't followed your meal plan, medication schedule, or exercise recommendations to the people who care about you. Guilt goes hand in hand with denial and dishonesty. It is so easy to say it like you wish it were instead of how it is. Practicing honesty in your relationships takes courage.

For 20 years Sarah answered her mother's predictable question, "How's your diabetes?" with "It's fine." One day she decided to tell her mother that diabetes and the foot problems it caused were not at

*all "fine." She explained how painful her feet were,
and for the first time, her mother knew how she
could help. A friend had raved about how helpful a
podiatrist had been, so she suggested that Sarah
call the podiatrist and that she would be happy to
go with her. Sarah had never considered seeing a
foot doctor and was touched by her mother's caring.*

Friends and loved ones need honest communication from you to
help you cope with difficulties. Building a relationship of mutual
respect depends on being honest. Working from accurate information will allow your doctor to really help. Health care professionals base their health care decisions on what you tell them. Honesty
is a crucial aspect of empowering them to do their jobs. Practicing
this may feel awkward at first, but it will encourage your doctor to
be honest and give the best care for your health needs.

Respecting limitations. Everyone is limited by how much they
can understand and how well they can respond. It is unfair to expect
anyone, including yourself, to do or to know it all. Sometimes
stopping to think about where another person is coming from and
about what s/he knows may prevent you from feeling
misunderstood and angry. The simple act of asking that person to
repeat and elaborate on his/her perceptions will give you the
opportunity to learn whether s/he see things the way you do. At
times you will not be able to persuade another person to share your
view. Respect this. Work at his/her level of understanding or
acceptance until s/he is ready to learn more. This prevents
frustration and wasted time.

Using feedback. You have the right and responsibility to ask for
clarification and assistance in fitting recommendations into your
life. Remember, no one can know what your life is like except you.
You do not have to accept what a health care provider or family
member advises, but you do have to decide what is best for you.
Keep in mind that the advice or feedback may not be what you want

to hear, but it still may be what you need. Your challenge is to listen to your inner wisdom and to make a decision of how to use the feedback. Using negotiation skills and taking the time to reflect on the feedback offered will help you determine what works for you.

The language of treatment and words of healing

How do you view your situation and how do you speak on your own behalf? The words that you and others use to describe your diabetes will affect how you feel about yourself and how others treat you. You may not be able to control the words others choose, but you can control what you do in response to them. One choice is to ignore them; another is to ask to be spoken to more respectfully. For example, after a brief visit with your physician, you hear her say to her nurse, "this brittle, insulin-dependent diabetic needs help with compliance and tightening her control. Could you arrange an appointment with our diabetes educator to review insulin and exercise regimens?" How would you feel? Some people might feel diminished. What could the doctor have said that would have made you feel supported?

Does your own choice of words influence how you view yourself and diabetes? Yes. Throughout the book we have used words that convey an attitude of respect, words that can fit into your vocabulary instead of those traditionally used to talk about diabetes. These words convey our respect for you. Your choice of words is powerful. It takes time, but using words that reflect your beliefs and values will set the stage for you to grow in the direction you want to go. Using affirmations, which is described in Chapter 8, is an excellent way to do this. The words you use convey not only what you are trying to say, but also your worldview and your expectations. The first step in improving your relationship with diabetes may be as simple as changing the words you use to discuss it.

The process of relating to others

Here are a few things worth considering about building and nurturing relationships.

Forming new relationships. Remember that your best friend used to be a stranger. Break the ice by introducing yourself and asking open-ended questions; this is the hardest part. A friendship may grow. Initially it's probably unnecessary to bring up diabetes, but trusting another person with this information tends to strengthen relationships. It is easier to bring it up when you are feeling good, instead of waiting until you have to bring it up. Relationships are strained when you withhold information that would help the other person understand you.

Sheila, a parent of a six-year-old, still can't talk to her daughter's new school teacher after running into her in a parking lot when her blood sugar was seriously low.

> *I* have this sinking feeling in the pit of my stomach when I think how confused she must have been. I didn't recognize her or follow her description of how wonderful Sarah was doing in her new class. I can't bring myself to tell her that I was having hypoglycemia. I am so embarrassed. She must have thought I didn't care.

Asserting yourself. Assertiveness may not come naturally to you. Respecting yourself is at the core of being assertive. Through practice, you will become less awkward. You can memorize assertive answers and practice them in the mirror. Don't fall into making excuses or apologizing. The first step is to know what you want from another person. The more clear you are in your own head, the easier it is to be assertive. You have to assert yourself as a woman and as a person with diabetes.

> *M*y friend Alice always chose the restaurant we went to after bingo on Fridays. Her favorite was Lou's Diner. This was a real problem because we always had to wait for a table. One night when we went out of the noisy bingo hall, I asked if we could go to Friendly's. She said, "Sure." Why did I wait so long?

Listening for the meaning behind the message. It takes time and attentiveness to hear what another person is saying to you. Listening to the words is the first step. Hearing the intended meaning involves much more. The tone of voice, facial expression, body language, and gestures all reflect add meaning. If you are unclear, ask for further explanations, and listen. Don't respond. Don't defend. The final step is to check with yourself to see how able you are to hear. Is your head too full of your own issues to listen objectively? You must be able to separate your own emotions and biases from his or hers. Your emotional and physical state will affect what you hear. Being aware of this contributes to clearer communication.

Methods of getting your message across. Say it over the phone. Announce it at a dinner date. Let him know on a long walk. Call her at work. Sing it. Write it. Fax it. E-mail it. There are many ways to convey a message. Choose a method that you are comfortable with and that suits the other person. This makes success more likely.

Negotiating for What You Need

Negotiation is what people do each time they make an agreement. From deciding what's for dinner to working out your diabetes treatment plan, people are making agreements. The way you handle the interaction that leads to the agreement is negotiation. Many things influence this, but there are some definite "people skills" that can help you arrive at agreements that suit your needs.

Conflict and the value of awareness
Deborah Jones, a trainer in negotiation and problem-solving skills, points out three common mistakes that can derail negotiations.

Being scared off or turned off by the other person's approach to the problem. You never get to the problem itself. Common ways of approaching a problem are: avoiding, accommodating, competing, compromising, or collaborating. Each has good and bad points. People tend to favor one or two of these under pressure, and there is almost always pressure coming from somewhere. Be aware of each other's styles. Mistrust of an approach may lead you to mistrust the person and derail the negotiation.

Forgetting to ask why we want what we want. You may know what you want, but do you know why you want it? Does the other person? Do you both have the same interests and goals? Try to avoid getting into a tug of war over options. Try to discuss the reasons *why* an option is the favorite one.

Not spending enough time discovering the differences between the two parties. Be willing to discover and discuss differences. Conflict is inevitable, and it is always an opportunity to learn something valuable. You need this information in order to change and grow. Try being creative instead of spending valuable time arguing over a solution.

Basic negotiating skills

Working with confusion and emotion
- Think through your goals for the relationship by asking yourself what would be right between you.
- Be "hard" on or angry at the problem and "soft" on the people involved. Separate the people from the problem.
- Reject insults. Firmly confront a verbal personal attack without leaving the negotiation. For example, "When you _____, I feel _____, which will only make it more difficult for us to succeed here/ solve the problem/ address your concern about _____."
- Ask yourself what you imagine (it may or may not be true) about this other person, and then ask what is causing you to imagine it. Say, "I see you _____, and that causes me to imagine _____. Is this true?"

Defining the needs of both people

- State the problem.
- State what your desire is, even though you are not sure how to achieve it at this point.
- Use active listening. Restate what you believe the person has said, that is, what he wants, his concerns, or his desires. Ask him to repeat to you his understanding of what you have said. Let him know how correct he is.
- Directed listening. State what you want, your concerns, and your desires.
- Clearly come to an agreement about what the problem is before either of you criticize or propose solutions.

Generating options—ideas to choose from

- Be firm on *interests* while being flexible about options.
- Stop the other person from mixing up the process of generating options with deciding among them.
- Explain that listening does not equal agreeing

Considering fairness

- Ask what she would do in your shoes.
- Ask her what she thinks would be fair in this situation. Find out why she feels that way.

Choosing among the options

- Reframing. Explain how the solution you like could be a good solution from his point of view, too.
- Reframing. Explain how the solution he likes could help you.
- After you have brainstormed a list, note the ones that help both of you. Could you live with any of the others as well?
- Make a final agreement specific enough so that both of you know exactly what to do and when.

Interacting with professionals

Viewing the professionals in your life as allies instead of gods will be relieving to both of you. You all have meaningful roles, limits, and areas of expertise. The practices below will inspire relationships that will serve your need for support and understanding and the professional's desire to help you. Your involvement in the relationship is very different from that with friends and family. You are seeking professional care and paying for it. The more you can do to find professionals you respect, who share your beliefs about health and health care, the easier it will be to communicate with them.

Finding a professional who fits your needs. Increasingly, insurance companies are determining who can take care of your medical needs and how. Their interest. like yours, is to keep you healthy. If you like the person who is taking care of you, and your insurance company asks you to change to another provider, find out who your representative is and ask whether your doctor can be included on their list of preferred providers. Ask to speak to the medical director or case worker who is most suitable to hear your case. This may not be possible, but don't give up easily. Persistence often pays off.

If you are not satisfied with your current relationship with your health care team, as with any other relationship, the best tactic is to share your concerns with them. This may feel awkward but does not need to be disrespectful. Providers expect to be questioned, even if they seem uncomfortable with it. First, you need to know what you need and what you want from the professional caring for you. Another tactic would be to seek out a different professional who can work with you.

Ideally, you will have one primary care physician who takes care of your general health needs and coordinates care with other specialists. This person should take the time necessary to talk with and listen to you, help you plan ahead to prevent problems, prescribe medications carefully, be available by phone, have your trust and respect, and know about all of your health problems. A provider's qualifications and interpersonal skills, the office location, and ease of scheduling appointments are also important for you to consider.

It is as impossible for your primary care physician to meet all your requirements. You need to prioritize them and understand the limitations set by who pays the bills (yourself, an insurance company, or the government) and find the best match available. At times, nothing else matters except the provider's ability to diagnose or treat your medical problems.

Preparing for a visit. Getting ready for a visit with your health care provider involves more than just deciding what to wear and how to get there. You need to be prepared to describe your concerns to her in ways she can understand. Taking the time beforehand to carefully review your reason for seeking their help. List your questions and concerns. Note what you think caused or influenced the problem, and other factors influencing it. This practice builds a relationship based on mutual respect and responsibility.

Understanding what they say. Hearing and understanding are two different acts. You need to take responsibility for requesting clear explanations from all health care providers. Ask them to tell you again, write it down, or tell it to a friend or family member. Getting over your pride when you can't follow what your health care provider is saying is the first step. They are not judging you; they are only trying to help.

Following through. Following through on the recommendations of your health care provider is always more difficult when you get home. The real challenge is to find ways to work the new requirement into your existing lifestyle. Consider consulting a diabetes nurse educator or a dietitian who are trained to help you problem-solve these issues.

Resources for getting the support you need

There are many ways to get the support you need from other sources. Here are a few of those sources.

Classes and support groups. Simply being with other people who are on the same diabetes pathway is enormously uplifting. Empathy and strategies from other people living with diabetes provide a kind of support found nowhere else. Find a group by calling local hospitals or the nearest American Diabetes Association chapter found in the white pages of your telephone book.

Books and magazines. Reading is one of the best ways to learn something new. There are many sources of information that can help you learn and grow. Look for information that is written and presented in ways you can easily understand. Ask support people for their advice on books that might help you. You may be amazed at how much has been written for people working on the same challenges that you are.

Agencies and organizations. There is a rich network of organized groups whose purpose is to offer assistance. Finding an agency to assist you takes some effort on your part. Agencies are more aware of each other than you probably are of them. So, asking one agency representative to suggest who else might offer assistance with a problem is a good idea. The phone book is a good place to start finding out about local and state agencies.

Health insurance providers. Insurance companies do a lot more than pay your medical bills. Read the literature they send you. Ask if they cover services such as health club membership discounts that may help you meet your wellness goals. You should have an insurance representative. It is that person's job to communicate with you about the services they offer and to resolve any problems you are having.

Socializing Through the Seven Ages of Womanhood

When you leave your nuclear family, your social network shifts from school, friends, and family to peers, co-workers, and authority figures in the greater community. Communicating with parents can be particularly difficult as they have to give up their responsibilities for your health care, finances, well-being, and diabetes management. Experimenting with ways of interacting with others will help you develop styles that fit your personality. The ways that diabetes influences your relationships with friends and lovers and how you respond to them shapes your self-concept.

> *My experiences at the hospital have taught me that there are caring people out there who understand how hard having diabetes is. Even if my family doesn't care, I know other people do.*

> *Diabetes is as much a part of me as the color of my eyes. If other people can't accept that, it's their problem.*

> *I am so afraid to tell Mike that I have diabetes. Things are going so well between us, I don't want to mess up our relationship now.*

As you settle into a new job, town, or living arrangement your relationships and social circles can change. Intimate friendships and a committed partnership can provide the social support that you need as you adapt and redefine your roles. Diabetes can burden you with financial and health decisions. It is challenging to make commitments (living arrangements, marriage, taking a job) and take on responsibilities (having children, paying bills, etc.). Relationships you can trust help you navigate through this stage. Your negotiation skills will be called on now to make agreements that work for you and are constructive for your relationships.

Once you have established (or reestablished) a place to live and adjusted to your multiple roles (single woman, teacher, mother, domestic engineer, writer), you may find yourself becoming less satisfied, bored, or burned out. Participating in women's or mother's groups, volunteering, or taking a class are good ways to meet people who share your challenges and responsibilities. Groups and friendships can provide support as you begin to raise questions about your roles, relationships, and responsibilities. Communicating with your partner, children, and co-workers so that your needs are valued is important as you redefine your roles and practice self-care. Having or developing diabetes at this stage highlights this need.

When job or child rearing responsibilities become less demanding, you're left with a mixed bag of emotions. On one hand, you may have more time and freedom. On the other hand, you have less to do and fewer people there for you. You may now have the time and be less driven to prove yourself, so you can risk making new friendships and spend more time on the ones you have. Your social network may expand as your creative interests blossom. Your need for friendships and social support grows with changes in family structure and increased time for social activity. Companionship in intimate relationships becomes more valued. Diabetes and other health problems may get in the way of you enjoying new freedoms or focusing on your priorities. Communicating and negotiating with health care providers gains importance.

Marge had always hated having to eat meals at regular times and chasing insulin reactions with high calorie snacks. She had heard about the new fast-acting insulin and decided to ask about it. Her physician agreed that it was a good solution. She went to a dietitian and learned to count carbohydrates and adjust insulin to work with her food and activity. She learned how to interpret patterns in her blood sugar levels and to make informed decisions about her insulin and food intake. Her whole life opened up with this new awareness. For the first time, since her diagnosis 5 years ago, she really felt in control. She regulated her blood sugars by matching the insulin with the meals that she ate. This gave her predictable blood sugar levels and a sense of freedom she never imagined possible. She even felt confident enough to travel to her sister's home in China, something she had not even dreamed of doing before.

Moving beyond child rearing and menopause can provide you a whole new sense of freedom. You'll probably review your personal, marital, and career goals at this time. You may find yourself feeling satisfied or dismayed with your life's accomplishments, and this will impact your self-esteem. Relationships with people who reinforce your strengths and accomplishments are particularly important at this stage.

Deepening wisdom in your later years can bring steadier commitments to yourself and others. Retirement can provide a new awakening to a marriage. You will grieve for loved ones who die and place increased value on other friendships, old and new. You will be challenged to enjoy and use your solitude creatively. The transformation of your social network through life changes such as retirement and death may propel you to seek new relationships and support. As always, relationships with people who reinforce your strengths are important as you cope with losses. Supporting others at this time will be very rewarding to you, too.

You may become more dependent on those who once depended on you. The quality of your past relationships becomes evident. Communication may be difficult. Your mature sense of perspective and ability to accept limitations promotes honest interactions and can heal and deepen relationships. Diabetes is no longer so difficult socially, yet the physical requirements demand more from your relationships than ever before. Getting your social as well as physical needs met, if you can no longer meet them yourself, may be your paramount challenge. Trusted friends and family who care for and communicate on your behalf is the ultimate gift of meaningful relationships.

Relating with your own needs in mind

Self-care does not end with what you eat, how you move, and what you do to care for your body. Relationships cultivated with regular loving attention improve your health and vitality and have even been shown to be the strongest predictor of longevity! It is often said that the "people" part of a job is the most challenging, yet it is the "people" that most of us miss when leaving a job. The work of living with diabetes is no different.

Chapter 5

Job Satisfaction: Enjoying Meaningful Experiences

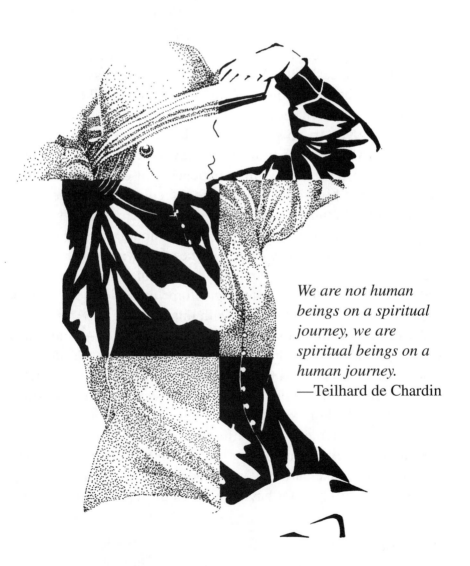

We are not human beings on a spiritual journey, we are spiritual beings on a human journey.
—Teilhard de Chardin

Diabetes and Your Body, Mind, and Spirit

Living with diabetes is not just a matter of numbers and physical events. It affects how you live in your body, use your mind, and experience yourself. Diabetes becomes another path to self-knowledge and connectedness.

Have you ever wondered just how much having diabetes influences who you are and how you act? Have you ever had a sinking feeling after a spat, thinking that maybe your blood sugar was to blame for your negative remarks? In the same way, women commonly question their emotions in relation to pre-menstrual syndrome (PMS) and menopause. You could say to yourself, "I am easily irritated, so I'll test my blood sugar. This is the way I tend to react when my blood sugar gets above 250." The more you learn to rely on your own internal wisdom, the easier it will be to experience wellness.

It takes practice. Getting to know your body is like getting to know what a newborn needs. First you look at and listen to the baby cry, and then you try to satisfy her with a diaper change, feeding, or rocking. After a lot of trial and error, you begin to notice subtle differences in her cries. With experience you develop a routine, meeting a loud high-pitched cry with a feeding and a quieter cry with a cuddle. In time you will be able to decipher your own body's language, whether it is sweaty palms, dry mouth, muscle tension, headaches, cramps, or low energy in the same way. Your responsibility is to stop, take a deep breath, and determine what the headache and muscle tension might be telling before you decide how to react.

Let's take some time to work with this.

As a woman with diabetes, you have a unique tool—your blood sugar—giving you insight into your body's messages. Your blood glucose level affects and will be affected by what you think, what you feel, and what you do. Often you will receive a clear message from your body. For example,

- your shoulders are tense after working long hours.
- after a week of fluctuating blood sugar levels, you are tired when you take care of your grandchildren.
- you are thirsty, after having high blood sugar for a few days.

Listening To Your Body

Rest with your eyes closed for a few minutes.

Scan your body and note if you feel any discomfort (tension, pain, swelling, tingling, or numbness). Focus on
- Your head (skull, eyes, ears, mouth, and nose) and neck
- Your shoulders
- Your chest
- Your arms and elbow joints
- Your wrists and fingers
- Your abdomen
- Your back
- Your bladder and ovaries
- Your pelvis
- Your legs and knees
- Your feet and toes

Go back to any areas where you noticed something and ask yourself, "What could this feeling be telling me?"

_____

_____

Ask yourself, "What can I do right now to take care of this?"

_____

_____

Ask yourself, "What could I do in the future to prevent or help me with this?"

_____

_____

Your initial reaction may be to ignore it. It is bothersome. In some instances it is healthy not to let discomfort slow you down. This is discipline. Other messages cannot be ignored (e.g., heart-attack symptoms) because they indicate that you are at immediate risk. Most messages are more subtle. Chronically ignoring these signs and symptoms can lead to serious problems down the road. You need a way to determine which bodily signs to respond to and when. This is a critical skill in diabetes self-management. By learning to understand what your blood sugar numbers mean in terms of signs and symptoms, you begin to gain a sensitivity that makes it easier to manage your diabetes and be well.

Writing down how your body feels when you know there has been a change—such as increased stress, low or prolonged high blood sugar levels, or during your monthly cycle—will teach you to notice the effect of this change on your body. This is awareness. Being aware of yourself is the basis of self-care, emotional strength, and spiritual connectedness. Only by listening to your body can your mind and spirit thrive.

Regard blood sugars as a barometer. They remind you to stop, listen, and reflect on what's going on inside you.

One woman says of her menstrual cramps, "They slow me right down and are a good reminder that I need to make some adjustments and tune in to the wisdom of my body." (In the House of the Moon: Reclaiming the Feminine Spirit of Healing, p. 82.)

Fluctuations in blood sugar can be viewed in the same way. High or low blood sugar certainly causes you to slow down. This opportunity for reflection is all too often missed by women. Instead, we tend to focus on guilt, worry, or frustration and hastily move on before we learn from the experience. The next time you experience a pattern of high or low blood sugar, reflect on what your body might be telling you. Ask yourself whether you are pacing yourself. Is this a signal to nurture your body? In what ways can living with diabetes serve you as a woman?

Women are taught to pay attention to external measures rather than to listen to internal messages. The measure of your success too often is reduced to weight, eating a low-fat diet, walking one mile at least three times a week, and maintaining blood sugar levels between 70 and 120. These external measures do give you information about what's going on inside you. But you need to decide what this information means to you and what to do in response to it. Yes, you are responsible for finding out the facts about what is healthy for you. You can get help from your health care team, health literature, supportive friends, and family.

As a girl of eight, Allyson sat at camp listening to a respected diabetes doctor explain that girls with diabetes should not plan on having babies due to the complications and potential birth defects. All her dreams of being like her mom were shattered. Years later, she decided to get pregnant anyway. Allyson read everything she could get her hands on about diabetes and pregnancy. She accepted her doctor's explanation that her delivery would have to be induced and could easily require a Cesarean section (C-section). She took birthing classes but paid little attention to the details of natural labor and delivery. Just as the blood sugar machine had helped her succeed with the pregnancy, the machine measuring her contractions and her baby's heartbeat told her how her labor was progressing. After 24 hours of induced, nonproductive labor, Allyson was thrilled for the doctor to perform a C-section and bring her healthy baby girl into the world. However, later she felt as though her experience of one of life's most vital moments was reduced to watching a machine and feeling like a statue from the waist down.

Three years later at a birthing center, Allyson had a different experience. She was coached to deliver naturally. She came to the induced delivery of her second child informed, involved, and confident that she could depend on her support team. Allyson was aware of the power of her body. She ignored the machines, paid attention to herself, and enjoyed the natural delivery of a healthy baby girl. Even if she had needed another C-section, Allyson was so much more involved with this birth that she knew she could handle it either way.

Allyson's first birth experience was shadowed by her fears from childhood. Those fears were calmed by watching the machines of medicine, but she was not as involved as she wanted to be with the birth of her daughter. She was thrilled to have a healthy baby but wanted a different experience the next time. With the second birth, she participated fully in the experience. She heard the messages her contractions communicated and responded with confidence, using the Lamaze skills she had learned. When the time came, she worked in harmony with her contractions to push Rachel into the world. She was in touch with this experience.

Pat had been on diets since she was 10 years old. After being told that she needed to lose weight, she fell into the cycle of yo-yo dieting. She went shopping for the latest low-fat, low-sugar junk foods and starved for a week, only to lose and regain the same eight pounds. Pat thought of her body only in terms of how much it weighed. She felt good when she lost weight, felt horrible when she gained, and didn't notice much else about her physical self. Pat avoided mirrors and didn't like looking at herself at all. She hated feeling so self-conscious and found herself staying at home more and more. Each weigh-in during her regular visits to her doctor seemed like judgment day. She always had a good reason for gaining the weight after losing it but still felt like a failure. Then, at the age of 56, Pat began to change. She gave up her desire to look like Marilyn Monroe. She cared less what she looked like and wanted to spend

*more time with friends and travel, now that she could.
A group of friends from church convinced her to join
their informal swimming group. Reluctantly, she went
and enjoyed being with friends, so she kept going. She
decided to join the local recreation department with a
friend, and after six months of swimming, she lost 17
pounds without really trying. Swimming felt good. She
began to notice that she didn't eat as much when she
spent more time doing things with her friends.*

If you strive to measure up to external standards, you must look outside to see whether you have succeeded. This invalidates you. When you trust yourself, and listen to your own wisdom, you can define and enjoy your own successes. You are your own authority. This is how to live a more connected and fulfilling life.

Consider Your Body

Your body is the tool you use to relate to the world. You modify it to work for you, and you adjust your life to fit its abilities. The way your body functions determines how you perceive and respond to all your experiences.

Every woman's body works in partnership with her mind and spirit to give meaning to her experiences and to determine how best to react to them. Diabetes can challenge your natural ability to see, feel, and hear. It also heightens your ability to pick up internal cues signaling conditions, such as infection, stress, or hormonal changes. Developing this ability to sense what is going on in your body will help you better understand what affects you. When you react to a cue, you will usually choose a reaction that promotes wellness. We seldom think that we can choose how to react. We think that a reaction happens too quickly for that, but there is time.

Having diabetes certainly influences what you choose to do with your body, such as running a marathon, traveling overseas, or having children. But so do many other things. Setting limitations on what you do with your body is part of taking care of yourself. Determining where to set these limits is tricky. It involves mediating between your desires, your physical and emotional comfort, and your beliefs about what is possible. So many times we decline opportunities for fun and recreation because we are afraid of what "they" think or because we think we can't do it. For instance, you might decline a request to dance because you don't want everyone looking at the way your body moves on the dance floor.

If you've never tried or are sure you have lost it physically, your self-imposed limitation can become rigid. You may be beyond even thinking of going for a swim or to a dance. The emotional impact of convincing yourself that you are unable to participate in things that are fun for you takes the spark out of life and the spunk out of you. How you think about your body is the basis of how you determine your own limits. And, generally, you can do more than you think you can!

Your Body

The abilities of my body that I can depend on include...

_____

I am fortunate to live in a body that...

_____

I am limited by my body because...

_____

If I could change one thing about my body it would be...

_____

Consider the answers given by Irene, 58, an avid gardener who worked in a local greenhouse. The abilities she could depend on include

> *...being able to lift almost anything and rarely getting even the slightest cold.*

She felt fortunate to live in a body that

> *...had great stamina allowing her to work long hours in her garden. She loved the time she spent there and enjoyed the extra income that selling vegetables provided.*

She felt limited by her body because

> *...her vision was affected by retinopathy, making it difficult to see at night. She hated not being able to go out to bingo the way she used to.*

She would like to change

> *...being tall. It had always been a difficult thing for Irene. She wondered if her height caused the osteoporosis that was beginning to affect her.*

What do you think about Irene? Can you see your body as clearly as you see hers?

Lets take a moment to look at how phenomenal your body is.

- The combined pulling strength of all the muscles in your body equals 25 tons.
- Your heart pumps the equivalent of 5,000 to 6,000 quarts of blood through you every day.
- Your ears can discriminate among more than 300,000 tones.
- Your brain, many times more complex than the most advanced computers, operates on the amount of electrical power that would light a 10-watt bulb.

- Your eyes can distinguish nearly 8 million differences in colors.
- The surface area of your lungs is 1,000 square feet—20 times greater than the surface area of your skin.
- Your bones manufacture 1 billion new red blood cells every day, replacing old ones at a rate of 1.5 million per second.
- Your circulatory system is more than 70,000 miles long.
- Your digestive tract is 30 feet long.
- One cubic inch of your bone can withstand a two-ton force.

—Lonny J. Brown, PhD, in *Self Actuated Healing*

This complicated structure you live in is a true miracle. Thinking for your pancreas is an amazing task to be given. Treated with respect and honor, your body could provide you with a lifetime of awe. Living each day so that your body organs and systems can operate at full potential sure makes more sense (and is more fun) than just following guidelines to get the right numbers on your HbA_{1c} lab report.

Consider Your Mind

Your mind works in harmony with your body and your spirit to make sense of it all. Through your body you experience the world. Feelings give you clues as to what these experiences mean to you and the importance they have in your life. Knowledge can help you interpret your experiences. Your spirit gives you perspective about these experiences in the world beyond what you can see.

The diagnosis of diabetes, onset of complications, an identity crisis, or the death of a loved one are all losses and are followed by the grief process. All of us grieve our losses. This is a normal adjustment to loss and the changes that result. The stages in the grief process have been defined by Elizabeth Kubler-Ross as denial, anger, bargaining, depression, and gradual acceptance. It is common to go back through previous emotional stages, when you have to work through new challenges or rework old ones. It is also common to get stuck in a stage of grief as you work through them. Seek professional help if you feel you are in trouble.

You also experience a wide variety of emotions related to living with diabetes every day. These range from elation to despair and are as unique as you are.

Check off the emotions you commonly feel in relation to having diabetes.

○ shock	○ sadness	○ fear	○ curiosity
○ anger	○ pride	○ boredom	○ nothing
○ depression	○ frustration	○ anxiety	○ happiness
○ deprivation	○ satisfaction	○ resentment	○ relief
○ gratitude	○ guilt	○ regret	○ balance
○ satisfaction	○ happiness	○ embarrassment	○ joy

In the box below is an exercise to help you examine your emotions about diabetes and the affect they have on your behavior. There are two steps to this exercise. Step one is to list the emotions you feel about the listed aspects of diabetes. Step two is to think about how each emotion causes you to react and write it down. For example, Audry feels angry after getting herself out to exercise and having serious insulin reactions each time. Her emotional response to exercise is anger. Her reaction is not to exercise.

List the emotions you feel in relation to the words listed below.

Emotions and Behavior

Word	Emotion	Resulting Impact On Your Behavior
A cure	_____	_____
Pancreas	_____	_____
Me	_____	_____
Meal plan	_____	_____
Blood sugar testing	_____	_____

Emotions and Behavior (continued)		
Word	**Emotion**	**Resulting Impact On Your Behavior**
Family support	_____	_____
Future complications	_____	_____
Current complications	_____	_____
Injections	_____	_____
Exercise	_____	_____
Pregnancy	_____	_____
Health insurance	_____	_____

Is there an overriding theme to the emotions you have listed? How do they influence what you think about yourself, what you feel, and what you do in response? What can you do to gain mastery over your emotions and not allow them to control how you react or behave? They can jeopardize the way you take care of yourself and interact with others.

Emotionally what we feel and believe about ourselves also colors our experience with life and life with diabetes. A woman who feels positive about herself is more likely to cope with the predictable crises and feel better than a woman who is fed by negative messages. (Look at the chart on the next page.)

Knowing and valuing who you are as a woman influences how you view your path and where it leads you. This is not to say that choosing a positive attitude ensures there will be no health problems. But it does enhance your ability to handle the problems as they arise without compromising yourself or your sense of integrity. The more you consider yourself as a priority, the more apt you will be to seek out assistance when you need it, follow through on your own good sense, and enjoy the feeling of well-being.

You Are What You Think

Positive self-image	Negative self-image
Acknowledge diabetes exists. "I am worth it." "I must take care of myself." ↓	Denial of disease. Shame, guilt, blame. ↓
Choose to adopt some healthy behaviors. ↓	Unhealthy behaviors. ↓
Handle the ups and downs. Move through the periods of sadness and discouragement. ↓	Negative thoughts about self or diabetes. Sabotage self-care efforts. ↓
Seek training to become more aware of choices and support during a difficult life challenge. "My needs and desires are important." ↓	Complain: "Why me? I can't do all this." Unhappy. ↓
Negotiate treatment strategies with the health care team. "I am uncomfortable with this meal plan. It doesn't work for me. I need something else." ↓	Isolation, pain, loneliness. "They just don't understand." Decreased energy for self-care. ↓
Encouragement: Feeling good about the small accomplishments. ↓	Discouraged: "It will never get better." ↓
Emotional and physical needs being met. ↓	Progressive physical or emotional health problems. ↓
Positive feelings about self.	Denial, shame, guilt. Negative feelings about self.

Consider Your Spirit

Your spirit encompasses all that gives your life real meaning. In her book *Living with Diabetic Complications,* Judy Curtis reminds us that having peace of mind rather than bodily health as our primary goal allows us to focus on what really matters. Peace of mind is something you do have the power to create and that is what really motivates you to take care of yourself. And taking care of yourself improves your physical health.

If your primary goal is peace of mind, you won't make yourself crazy trying to be perfect. When you are in touch with what really matters, you are motivated to do the work that is necessary to achieve and maintain wellness. For example, getting the best care during pregnancy is motivated by the desire to ensure the health of the baby. Regular exercise and attention to blood sugar management is motivated by wanting to feel well enough to do all your jobs. Or you may be motivated to make better food choices, not by weight control, but by a desire to see your grandchildren grow up.

One way to connect with your spirit is through listening to your inner voice. This voice is influenced by the messages we internalize from ourselves and others. Meditation, exercise, prayer, and worship are ways women quiet themselves to connect with and strengthen this voice. Positive affirmations or self-talk are important ways to feed your soul. This process of listening to your inner wisdom gives you a foundation for making decisions, dreaming, and planning for the future.

Job Satisfaction

Your dreams for the future have a better chance of coming true when you have a vision of what you want to do and a sense of your abilities and talents.

Stop and think where you want to be. Ask yourself, "Am I doing what it takes to get there?" and "Am I giving myself positive messages to support my commitment and intentions of being well?"

What Really Matters to You?

List the things you most like to do or the activities that have the most meaning to you.

_____

_____

Complete the following sentences by writing down the first thing that comes to mind after reading them.

1. Life would hardly be worth living if it weren't for...

_____

2. If I could change one thing about my life at this point, it would be...

_____

3. I keep myself alive and energized by...

_____

4. What I like best about myself is...

_____

5. I feel most powerful when...

_____

6. I feel discouraged about life when...

_____

7. The one thing I want to do with my life is...

_____

8. To do this, I need to take care of...

_____

You have the ability to reframe the perception that diabetes is a disaster or that it limits you. You can be whole spiritually, emotionally, physically, and socially. The daily challenges of diabetes can teach us how to become whole.

Chapter 6

Adaptability: Embracing the Physical Challenges of Your Career

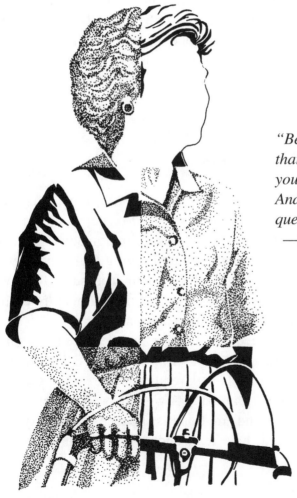

*"Be patient with all that is unresolved in your heart
And try to love the questions themselves."*
—Rainer Marie Rilke

In your quest for wellness, you need to pay attention to your general health and to the unique factors that put you at risk for developing long-term health problems. As a woman with diabetes, you are more likely to experience some health problems than are your friends who do not have diabetes. Your risk may be greater for developing early heart disease, osteoporosis, and impaired sexual function. You may experience some unique struggles during menopause. Having diabetes may also affect your experience with menstruation and pregnancy.

As part of your career in managing life as a woman with diabetes, you must be aware of how diabetes and your physical health are intertwined. You have choices to make in your diabetes management that will affect your general health. The good news is that you are not alone. This chapter tells you about these health risks and gives you ways to prevent or deal with the challenges you might encounter. Part of your success depends on including yourself at the top of your list of priorities. Taking care of your physical health, including diabetes, requires tender loving care. Remember, you are worth it!

Dealing With the Demons

To take care of your physical health, you may have to confront the issues that make it difficult for you to do what you need to do. Let's refer to these issues as the demons. Common demons are others' expectations of you, your own underlying fears and feelings of guilt, and an intimidating health care environment. To be successful in your quest for health, you will need a healthy attitude and a positive strategy to tame these demons.

If a woman is to succeed in managing her diabetes and keeping her whole being healthy, she needs time to herself. The time and energy that she needs for self-care require her to learn how to say "no" to others and feel OK about it. A woman is also likely to confront powerful feelings and emotions as she faces the reality of her physical health. She may have fears and feelings of guilt. Doubting her ability to cope with a health problem, she may put off dealing with it. She may feel that she caused the health problem and berate herself with statements like "I am bad." "If only I had done what I was supposed to do."

All people with diabetes are concerned about complications. So much energy is lost worrying about this unknown. It mobilizes some people to take charge and sometimes even to overdo. It paralyzes others, limiting their ability to enjoy life, take risks, and take care of themselves.

> *Chris, a woman with long standing diabetes, shared her experience of living with diabetes. So much of her early life with diabetes was spent living in fear and resentment. She said that she wasted a lot of energy worrying about complications and convinced herself that she could never live with those complications! This preoccupation sometimes paralyzed her, limiting her ability to take care of herself and consuming a great deal of energy, which prevented her from enjoying what the day presented to her. When she shared her story with us, Chris was living successfully with the complications of renal disease and total blindness. She said that all her worries had done her no good. In fact, she lives her life more fully now, despite these limitations. She has learned about her strengths and weaknesses through facing diabetes and her complications. This knowledge has calmed her and shown her the way to enjoy her life.*

Take-home message:
"You are worth the time it takes."
"Take the time to do what you need to do for yourself."
"Do not continue to live in fear. You will waste precious energy and life will pass you by. And if, just if, that which you feared most does happen, you will find a way to deal with it and still be whole."

Some people ask, "Why can't a woman be like a man or be treated like a man?" This issue surfaces for many people when they deal with the medical community. A woman is more likely to have her complaints treated by health care providers as though they were the result of PMS, postpartum blues, or depression, which may overlook other physical ailments. This may be due, in part, to the fact that women are more emotional when they communicate. The provider may not be prepared to handle this or have the time to allow the woman to express her whole story. Men are listened to differently because they tend to be less emotional and more matter-of-fact in their communications.

Moreover, a woman's complaints may not concern the provider because her symptoms do not necessarily match the symptoms or disease progression that the provider has been trained to expect. Until the Nurse's Health Study, which started in the 1980s, all research health studies were of men. This means that the lists of symptoms and treatment approaches that have been tested apply to men and may not always be right for women. This phenomenon has been referred to as the Yentl Syndrome. As more studies include women, physicians may became more sensitive to the differences between women and men.

Take-home message:
"You can communicate your needs and be understood by your health care provider."
"Do not give up trying. Figure out what you want to say and say it." "Believe in yourself."

Guiding Principles in Caring for Your Physical Being

Here are some ideas to keep in mind as you work on your health and wellness.

First, remember that it is never too late to start paying attention to yourself. You can always succeed at achieving a sense of wellness. Forgive yourself for the past. Focus on today. What do you want out of life? You may not be able to get rid of your health problems today, but you may be able to prevent them from getting worse. You can feel better. Recall Anna in Chapter 1. Wellness is not defined by the absence of disease. Wellness is a state of honoring who you are just as you are—having a sense of peace and respect, even for the illness part of yourself. Today is a fresh new start. Seek out new ways of reaching your goals in life. Chapter 8 will provide you with more ideas on how to do this.

Second, remember that your physical body may not always cooperate with your wishes and efforts. It can be very discouraging not to lose weight after working hard to follow a meal plan and exercise program. The body is complex. Sometimes what happens is not in your control.

Third, even though you cannot change your genetic makeup or control what happens, you do not have to give up. You can increase your chances of success by trying new approaches to keeping your body and mind as healthy as possible. Consider brainstorming new approaches or seeking support for your current approach with your health care provider, a nurse educator, or a friend.

Fourth, learn to listen to what your body is telling you. For example, if your blood glucose fluctuates, your weight changes, or your skin begins to dry out, stop and reflect on what your body needs. These symptoms may be telling you that you need to rest more, take time out for a refreshing walk, or drink more fluids. You may also hear your inner voice suggesting that the symptoms you have might mean a serious health problem. Work with your health care provider to distinguish real from imagined problems.

This whole book is about making choices and how to get better at identifying and taking care of your needs. You know that you can choose to ignore or to respond to these messages. You can ignore messages that your body is unhealthy. You can choose to turn to some addiction that will divert your attention, such as alcohol, overeating, or working excessively. Do you recall our discussion in Chapter 1? We explored how ignoring or denying your reality can lead to disharmony and "dis"ease. On the other hand, you can choose to listen to the messages and do something to take care

of the problem. For instance, you may finally go to the ophthalmologist to see how serious your visual problems are or to the psychologist to face the painful memories that limit your feelings of
self-worth. Facing things that are difficult or painful does undoubt-
edly force you to discover your own strength. This is the way your
soul grows. This helps you become stronger and healthier.

Fifth, learn how to communicate your needs or experiences
clearly and briefly. Practice with a friend stating what you feel your
problems are and asking for what you need to make you feel better. The other person may not always agree with your requests. Do
not take disagreement as a sign that your presentation or request
is not understood or important. Be prepared to discuss your position and be open to hearing the other person. Chapter 4 provides
you with more specific ideas for communicating on the job.

Sixth, believe in your own healing abilities. Many people believe
that women are natural healers. Our ancestors were shamans, mid-
wives, and healers of the sick. Reach for the inner healer within
you and get to know her. Learn to trust the wisdom and messages
from your own body and reclaim your power. Actively participate
in your own health. Learn to put your needs near or at the top of
your list of priorities.

Seventh, seek a health care provider or team of providers who
are able to work in partnership with you, who consider it their
responsibility to help strengthen your innate healing ability. Such
a partnership means the health care provider is the advisor who
evaluates your health and health risks, informs you of treatment
options, and explores with you how to apply the treatment options.
You must communicate your needs, concerns, and symptoms as
they surface and commit yourself to following the health plan you
and your health care provider designed. Consider setting up an
annual appointment with your providers to explore and confirm
what is happening with all parts of you. This is like spending time
creating an annual budget for your household or business. It is just
as important! You need to be aware of your health assets and your
limitations as you begin to prioritize how you will spend your precious time and energy.

The rest of this chapter gives you some ideas to explore with your health care provider.

Celebrate Being a Woman

One of the most important experiences in a woman's life is to express her sexual desires and give and receive pleasure. A woman's ability to experience her sexuality is influenced by how she perceives her own worth and physical abilities. She also needs a partner who is sensitive and caring.

Some women define sexuality as the ability to bear children. This definition tends to devalue the whole woman. It ignores how important it is to feel fulfilled by the intimacy, pleasure, and satisfaction of two people connecting with each other. Therefore, sexuality is as important to a woman in her 60s as it is to a woman in her 30s. Women with diabetes can have a healthy and sexually fulfilling life. However, many fear rejection or the negative consequences of future complications.

All too often we have heard women proclaim that they feel less attractive or appealing because of their diabetes. A woman is naturally concerned about the effect her diabetes will have on her ability to perform sexually and to satisfy her partner. The older woman who has recently developed diabetes might struggle with the fear that she will be rejected by her lifelong partner. Single and younger women also share this fear. Having low blood sugar on a date or during sexual intercourse can be devastating to the woman who has not discussed the potential for this to happen with her partner.

Unfortunately, experiences like these will often leave a woman feeling reluctant to develop an intimate relationship. How many times have you thought, "Will he think I am attractive once he knows I have diabetes?" "Will diabetes interfere with my ability to have a healthy sex life?" "Will I be a burden to my partner if I have complications?" No matter what your internal dialogue has been in the past, we hope that you will begin to believe in yourself and that your sexuality need not be lessened because of diabetes.

Sexual activity involves physical exertion and can result in a low blood sugar. When anticipating having sex, a woman may want to consider reducing the appropriate insulin. Or she can choose to eat something before having sex. For example, Shelly keeps a supply of raisins near her diaphragm. This makes it easy for her to eat some without having the moment of passion interrupted. If low blood sugar does occur, a woman may find that she is unable to perform as usual and cannot enjoy the experience. For another woman, being low may enhance her feelings of pleasure. It is important not to ignore the symptoms and to treat them as soon as it is reasonable. It will be important to discuss with your partner the potential for low blood sugar, the symptoms, and the treatment. Remember, you don't have to be alone with your diabetes.

Challenges to Sexual Health

A woman's sexual experience is influenced in part by the function and health of nerve fibers and blood vessels that feed the female genitals—the clitoris, vaginal wall, and vulva. Complaints of pain or decreased lubrication during intercourse or decreased sexual desire are common symptoms of sexual dysfunction in all women. Estrogen therapy may help improve lubrication. Using lubricants, learning to relax the muscles around the vagina, or trying different positions may help reduce pain during sex. If a woman has nerve damage, she may lose some sensation around the genital area. This can lessen her sexual arousal and pleasure.

Persistent high blood glucose levels can increase a woman's chance of vaginitis (inflammation of the vagina) or yeast infections. If you have problems with unusual discharge from the vagina, itching, or yeast infections, you should consult with your doctor to determine the best treatment for correcting the problem and improving your blood glucose control. High blood sugars can also sap a woman's energy and sense of vitality. Feeling sluggish and tired can interfere with how attractive and receptive one is to engaging in sexual activity.

Being able to enjoy the wide range of physical and emotional feelings associated with sexual contact is linked to the emotional state of the woman. Lack of trust in her partner or in her own ability can interfere with a woman's enjoyment. Likewise, poor communication between partners, depression, shame, or a poor self-image may interfere with a woman's sexual desire. Seeking help from a mental health professional can be very helpful in dealing with these issues.

Women who have multiple health problems may be taking medications that interfere with their ability to have fulfilling sexual contact. Some medications can interfere with a woman's libido (desire for sex). Others cause drying of the vaginal tissue, which leads to painful intercourse. If you are concerned, be sure to ask your doctor about the effects of your medications on your sexual health.

If you find that you are unhappy or concerned about the sexual area of your life, do not feel ashamed or alone. It may not be easy to communicate these concerns to your partner or to your provider. Yet, if you are to honor yourself as a woman and this is an issue for you, take the risk.

Monthly cycles

If you are still menstruating, you may have noticed your blood sugar values are higher around or during your monthly period. Blood sugar is affected by the natural release of hormones that cause your body to be more resistant to its own insulin or to insulin that you inject. Normally, blood sugar remains high for three to five days and gradually returns to the level it was before your period. Some women notice this change right before their monthly cycle. Others notice it during or right after. Each woman's body is different.

Your blood sugar can rise as a result of giving in to food cravings before the monthly cycle. During PMS or menstruation, you might have less energy and not want to exercise. If you stop exercising, your blood sugar may rise even higher. Your ability to control those cravings and to continue with your exercise program will help you balance your blood sugar.

It is important to discuss with your health care provider how to adjust your diabetes medication or treatment program during this time to keep blood sugar levels close to the desired target. Many women choose to ignore this temporary rise in blood sugar. This really isn't the best choice because elevations over time increase your chance for developing health problems and leave you feeling poorly as a result.

To determine the effect of your cycle on diabetes control, check your blood sugar two to four times a day the week before, during, and after your cycle for two to three months. Work with your health care provider to identify your individual blood sugar patterns in response to changes in hormone levels. This is a great time to also note the effect of alcohol and caffeine intake. Keep a log of your blood sugar, emotions, and intake of fat, carbohydrates, alcohol, and caffeine. Record when you feel better and worse. Explore with your doctor how to make changes in your medication schedule. Don't forget the positive effects of physical activity, relaxation techniques, and healthy nutrition!

Women with uncontrolled blood sugar may also have irregular monthly cycles and acne. Persistent high blood sugar may interfere with the release of hormones responsible for your menstrual cycle.

Contraception

If you have not experienced natural or surgical menopause (total hysterectomy), you will need some form of contraception, no matter how old you are or what type of diabetes you have. It is particularly important for a woman with diabetes to plan her pregnancy in order to give her baby the most healthy start.

Decisions about the best contraceptive methods should be made with your partner and your physician. Your health care provider will help you make this decision after taking into account your overall health, which method offers the best protection with the fewest side effects, and which one you are most likely to use consistently. You can find out more about contraception methods by talking to your health care provider and checking the resources listed later in this chapter. It is important to choose the right method that works for you! The purpose of this section is to highlight the issues you need to be aware of as they relate to your diabetes.

Contraception options range from abstinence to the pill. The method that is reliable and that helps prevent an unplanned pregnancy as well as an infectious disease is the best choice. The pill refers to a variety of oral contraceptives made from synthetic forms of two hormones involved with regulating the menstrual cycle, progestin and estrogen. A combination estrogen and progestin pill is slightly more effective than progestin alone (99% as compared to 98% success rate). In the past, a woman with diabetes was advised not to take the pill for two reasons. First, taking oral contraceptives could worsen her blood sugar control. In some instances, even today, a woman may find this to be true. She and her doctor will need to adjust her diabetes treatment program accordingly or she and her partner will have to agree on other options. Second, she may be at risk of developing problems with circulation and clotting, such as heart attacks or stroke. As the dose of estrogen and progestin has been decreased in newer pills, so has the risk for these problems.

However, women on the pill who smoke are at greater risk for circulation problems. Smoking causes the blood vessels to narrow, the walls of the vessels to thicken, and the blood to clot. That's why it is important for a woman to quit or reduce her smoking as much as possible. High HbA_{1c} levels or being dehydrated may also increase the chances of having blood clotting problems.

It is important for a woman on the pill to have her blood fats and blood pressure checked routinely. If you have high blood pressure or high blood fats (hyperlipidemia), you may need to use a different method of contraception. Taking the pill when you have high blood pressure can increase the chance that eye or kidney disease will get worse. The pill can also cause a rise in blood fat levels (cholesterol, LDL, and triglyceride levels). If you are concerned, speak to your doctor.

Side effects from the pill, such as weight gain, irritability, or break-through bleeding are reasons many women stop taking the pill. These side effects are more common with progestin-only pills. If you experience any discomfort with taking any oral contraceptive, it is important to discuss other options with your provider. For the best results, keep your diabetes under reasonable control, take the pill as prescribed, and inform your health care provider when you have side effects.

An Intrauterine Device (IUD) may be an attractive option for the woman who is past child bearing, is not likely to have any more children, and now has a single sex partner. In the past, women were discouraged from using the IUD because of the risk for pelvic infection or trauma to the uterine wall. The newer IUDs are considered to be far less likely to cause infection and undesired trauma. The IUD is an effective contraceptive method because it irritates the uterine wall making it difficult for the egg to get implanted. They may also be an effective choice because they do not affect blood glucose and blood fat levels.

Other barrier methods such as the diaphragm or condoms with spermicidal foam or gels, when used properly are effective methods that do not affect glucose control. The diaphragm is a rubber cap that the woman lubricates with a spermicidal gel and fits into her vagina and over her cervix before intercourse. It acts as a barrier to prevent sperm from entering the uterus. The uterus is where eggs are fertilized by the sperm. This is why it is called a barrier method of birth control. When used correctly, it can be up to 95% effective in preventing pregnancy.

Some women find the diaphragm awkward and difficult to use. They fear the loss of spontaneity in lovemaking. Because it can be inserted as much as an hour before intercourse, a little planning ahead will allow you to have some level of spontaneity. If you choose a diaphragm, it is important that your doctor fit it properly. Also, make sure he or she explains how to use it correctly. When women with diabetes use the diaphragm, they may have more yeast infections than women without diabetes.

Another barrier method of birth control is the condom, a thin membrane sheath that fits over the penis. It can be used effectively by itself, but it is even more effective when combined with a sperm-killing foam or vaginal gel suppository. Statistics show that when the condom and foam are used together, they are up to 85% effective in preventing pregnancy.

The major problem with barrier methods of birth control, such as the condom, is that they require some planning for use. They must be used every time intercourse occurs, and they must be used correctly. If not, they won't be effective.

The use of implantable contraceptive agents, such as Norplant, and those requiring routine injection by your doctor, such as Depo-Provera, are other alternatives for women with diabetes. They will affect blood sugar levels. Norplant is a small capsule with medication in it that is placed under the skin on the arm. This capsule releases small amounts of the medication over a long period of time, approximately 5 years. It must be surgically removed. Depo-Provera must be injected by your doctor every three months. This is not the method of choice if you do not keep your appointments. Both methods need to be combined with a condom to prevent sexually transmitted diseases.

No matter what method you choose, be sure you have informed your diabetes care provider about your contraceptive choice as this may affect your treatment plan.

Pregnancy

Thousands of women with diabetes have healthy pregnancies and healthy babies when they keep blood sugar levels as close to normal as possible before and during the pregnancy. If you are contemplating having a child, you, too, with the best care can expect a healthy pregnancy. You will want to prepare for the pregnancy and to work with a team of professionals who are experienced and comfortable working with a woman with diabetes. Usually this team will consist of, at a minimum, a diabetes doctor, a high risk obstetrician, a nurse educator, and a dietitian.

Ideally, a woman should plan for her pregnancy three to six months before she gets pregnant. You are looking for an HbA_{1c} within normal ranges. This level indicates that your diabetes is well managed and the risk of birth defects is low. The pre-pregnancy phase is also a good time to polish your diabetes self-management skills as well as have your overall health evaluated. A healthy mom increases the chances of having a healthy baby!

During pregnancy you will need to monitor blood glucose levels at least four times a day and to check your urine for ketones. You need to be prepared to make appropriate adjustments in your meal plan or insulin program, treat low blood sugar, and handle sick days. Working with a nurse and dietitian will help you learn these skills and more about how your diabetes will change during pregnancy.

Managing diabetes during pregnancy can be a challenge. The first three months are the most important to the development of the fetus. This is the time when the brain, nervous system, and body organs are developing. During this time, your blood sugar levels will change dramatically in response to hormone changes in your body and to morning sickness. Exhaustion and vomiting may further interfere with your ability to pay attention to your needs. Hormones released from the placenta during the second and third trimester make your body more resistant to insulin. You may be less sensitive to changes in blood sugar levels and to signs of hypoglycemia.

To help you plan your pregnancy, use the list below. Every woman should have the following areas evaluated before she gets pregnant. Your health care providers will help you determine when it is safe to become pregnant. Shop around for a health care team that will work well with you.

Before getting pregnant, have the following evaluations done and discuss with your provider their influence on whether or when to get pregnant.

- Eye evaluation with an ophthalmologist
- Blood pressure
- HbA_{1c} (overall blood glucose control)
- Kidney test for protein
- Presence of hypoglycemia unawareness (inability to detect low blood sugar)
- Presence of heart disease or other circulatory problems
- Breast and pelvic exams, Pap smear

Pregnancy can be an exciting and scary time. Learning and preparing as much as you can before getting pregnant will make a big difference for both you, your family, and your baby.

Lactation

Breastfeeding helps a new mother bond with her baby and enhances the baby's immune system, too. This can be a special and wonderful experience. It can also be challenging. Some infants take more time than others to learn how to latch on to the breast and to suckle, resulting in painful nipples, a frustrated mom, and an unhappy baby. Working with a supportive health care team will help you become confident and successful at breastfeeding your baby.

Women who choose to breastfeed may experience low blood sugar that occurs more often than before they were pregnant. The sugar levels drop as the baby feeds on the mother's milk. Some women report that their symptoms of low blood sugar change as well. It is possible to prevent frequent and severe low blood sugar through education and dietary counseling. Sugar or glucose tablets should be kept close by during feedings. You may need extra calories before, during, and after feeding the baby. Snacking or reducing the appropriate insulin will be important. This is particularly true to cover bedtime and night feedings.

Target ranges for your glucose control may be raised because you may experience low blood sugar in a more unpredictable fashion. It is also important to drink plenty of fluids and take in enough vitamins, minerals, and protein. Drinking a beverage each time you breastfeed is a good practice. Lactating women need 1,200–1,500 mg of calcium a day.

Menopause

In a previous section, we described how a woman's comfort with intimacy and her sexual expression are related to her physical and emotional health. She is also influenced by society's ideas of what female sexuality should be. Menopause is yet another female process that is colored by society's expectations and perceptions. Calling it "the change" leaves many people with an image of a woman transforming into an odd, irrational being. There is nothing odd about menopause nor about the woman who is menopausal.

So what is menopause? As a woman matures, her body goes through a predictable change, the climacteric, and the end of menstruation, called menopause. This normal process helps women make the transition from the age of childbearing and self-discovery to the age of wisdom and self-reflection. In some cultures, menopausal and post menopausal women are regarded as having power and insight that is of great value to the community. In our society women are confronted with the attitude that menopause is a medical disease signaling a deficiency and an end to their sexuality and value.

Menopause marks the ending of a woman's monthly menstrual cycle. It does not mean that she is no longer a sexual being. We all know a woman's worth and sexuality are not defined by her ability to have children. There are many women in their 50s, 60s, 70s, 80s, and even 90s who remain strong, attractive, and vital. During this time of self reflection, a woman comes into her own power. As author and teacher Caroline Myss points out, the post menopausal woman tends to feel less bound to society's expectations and approval. She often feels freer to make choices and to engage in relationships that are mutually fulfilling. This can be a time of celebration!

Women experience menopause differently. Your experience will be influenced by your physical health, your attitudes and fears about menopause, and the thoughts and beliefs of your friends. Some women experience relief knowing that they cannot get pregnant. Others grieve the loss of being able to have a child. Dr. Susan Love refers to menopause as puberty in reverse, wild with unpredictable swings in hormones and emotions. One month the estrogen levels are high, the next month they are low. Swings in hormones can cause difficulty sleeping, mood swings, and foggy thinking.

The symptoms experienced during menopause can often be confused with the symptoms of low and even high blood sugar. Hot flashes, moodiness, and short-term memory loss can be mistaken as a low blood sugar when, in fact, it is related to shifts in hormone levels. It is important for you to check your blood sugar before assuming that it is low and eating unnecessary calories. You may also see wide swings in glycemic control as the levels of hormones change or as a result of inadequate sleep.

During menopause, women often report low blood sugars that are stronger and more frequent, especially during the middle of the night. Sleep is often disrupted. Controlling diabetes can be very difficult. Just as it is during adolescence. Teenagers experience unpredictable swings in blood sugar because the levels of hormones like estrogen and growth hormone change frequently in a day's time. When the hormone levels increase, the blood sugar does as well. When the levels subside, blood sugar goes down. The same is true during menopause. Dealing with feelings of moodiness and fatigue or with the unpredictability of hot flashes and fluctuations in blood sugar can leave a woman feeling isolated, frustrated, and sad.

When your diabetes is difficult to control because of the changes in hormones, try to reduce the number of variables that affect your blood sugar level. Being more attentive to following your meal plan and management schedule is a good idea. Also, you will want to get adequate sleep and try relaxation techniques to help balance the effects of emotional and physical stress. So, nap when you need to and learn to breathe deeply! Try to be less critical of yourself during this time of transition. Be open to the new sides of yourself that will emerge. If you find yourself discouraged, you may want to consider approaching them with the attitude of one 16-year-old in response to her challenges with puberty. "It must be those HORMS!" This humor and lighthearted approach is refreshing and healthy! It is important to talk to other women with and without diabetes about their experiences to find out that you are not alone!

As the levels of estrogen and progesterone decrease, the body will be less resistant to insulin. Some women experience more hypoglycemia. You may find that you need to decrease the dose of your insulin or diabetes pills during or after menopause. Other body changes that you may see during and after menopause are vaginal dryness, resulting in painful intercourse, or increased risk for urinary tract infections. Persistent high blood sugar levels can make these conditions worse. Creams and gels can be used during sexual activity. Prompt treatment of vaginal and urinary tract infections is important.

If any of these symptoms interfere with your ability to complete your daily responsibilities or cause you undue stress, explore treatment options with your health care provider. Hormone replacement therapy (HRT) is an option for some women. A more detailed discussion of HRT can be found at the end of this chapter. Good nutrition, weight training, aerobic exercise, and adequate sleep form a foundation for a healthy transition during menopause. Because stress can make the symptoms worse, a woman may want to consider yoga, meditation, and other stress reduction techniques to help relieve the symptoms and enhance her overall well-being.

You may want to see a dietitian to review your needs for calcium supplements and to make changes to your meal plan. Some women report that calcium supplements help to reduce headaches, irritability, depression and insomnia. Calcium can be found in high amounts in dairy products, broccoli, cauliflower, pinto and soybeans, and nuts such as brazil nuts, hazel nuts, and almonds. The daily requirements for women before menopause is 1,000 mg of calcium. Postmenopausal women need 1,000 mg if they are on estrogen replacement therapy, and 1,500 mg if they are not. Some women report success using a higher soy diet and supplementing with bioflavinoids. If you choose to supplement with herbs, be aware that herbs are like medicines and should be taken under the supervision of someone trained in this area.

Matters of the Heart

For decades people have believed that women are not at risk for developing heart disease until they have gone through menopause. This is not necessarily true, especially for women with diabetes. As a woman with diabetes, you are at risk for developing heart disease earlier than your friends without diabetes. It is believed that estrogen provides a certain degree of protection against heart disease. Estrogen, released from the ovaries, helps to increase the production of HDL cholesterol, the good cholesterol, and to break down LDL cholesterol, the bad cholesterol. It also relaxes the smooth muscle of the blood vessels. Once a women experiences menopause, the production of estrogen goes down.

Diabetes negates the effects of estrogen. This means that no matter what age you are, you must pay attention to reducing your individual risk factors. Diabetes puts you at risk for heart disease and suffering from a life-threatening heart attack! If you do have heart disease, please check with your provider what your target blood sugar range should be. It is generally recommended to avoid hypoglycemia because of the increased chance of having a heart attack. Glucose ranges of 100–150 mg/dl may be best.

Symptoms of heart disease

Heart attacks occur when the heart muscle doesn't get enough oxygen. This can be a life-threatening event, especially for a woman with diabetes. Knowing the symptoms of a heart attack is important. However, you need to know that people with diabetes may not always feel these symptoms. Diabetes can damage the nerves that would normally warn you of a serious heart problem. So it is very important that you do not ignore any suspicious feelings! It is better to be seen by your doctor and find out that it is nothing than to let it go.

A list of the symptoms of heart attack is given in the box on the next page. Your symptoms of a heart attack may be very different from a man's, and they may be misinterpreted by the medical community. Symptoms common to women are marked with an asterisk. If you are concerned that you are experiencing a heart attack, be persistent and make your needs known. You should expect at a minimum a physical exam, blood work, and an electrocardiogram. In the second box is a list of additional symptoms or signs that a person with diabetes might experience.

Knowing what puts you at risk

Doing what you can to prevent heart disease is the first step. We realize that this is not always possible. You may have already had heart disease before you were diagnosed with diabetes. Even if you have heart disease, this section will help you try and prevent it from getting worse.

Classic Symptoms of Heart Attack
• Shortness of breath • Pain or tightness in your chest wall, jaw, or back of neck or down the right or left arm • Aching, throbbing, or a squeezing sensation* • Weakness, fatigue or drowsiness* • Hot poker tab between the chest* • Feeling like the heart jumps into the throat* • Heartbeat feeling like it is racing or skipping*
Additional Symptoms
• Blood sugar values suddenly out of control • Vomiting • Confusion • Extreme fatigue *common to women

Researchers are not clear about why women with diabetes have more heart disease. But because you have diabetes, you are more likely to have abnormal blood fat levels, problems with clotting, and high blood pressure than are your friends without diabetes. Any risk factor is more dangerous for the woman with diabetes. If you have high blood pressure, your chance of having heart problems is much greater than that of your friend who also has high blood pressure. High blood pressure and smoking is a very dangerous combination for a woman with diabetes! Let's look at the factors that put you at risk for developing heart disease. They are listed in the box below. Notice that being overweight is not at the top of the list. If you are overweight but all of the other risk factors are controlled or you are physically fit, your risk for heart disease is not that high.

Risk Factors for Heart Disease for the General Public

- Family history of heart disease
- Smoking
- High blood pressure: greater than 130/85 mmHg
- High cholesterol: greater than 240 mg/dl
- High triglycerides: greater than 130 mg/dl
- LDL cholesterol: greater than 130 mg/dl
- Cardiac risk ratio: greater than 3.5 for women
- Sedentary lifestyle
- Overweight (greater than 120% over desired weight)

A cardiac risk ratio is the way of determining how likely you are to have a heart attack soon. Ask your doctor to help you calculate and interpret your own cardiac risk ratio. Use the equation below. A number of 3.5 or below means that your risk is low. A score of 6 or higher means that your risk is very high and you should see your health care provider soon!

$$\text{cardiac risk ratio} = \frac{\text{cholesterol level}}{\text{HDL level}}$$

Example: If cholesterol is 210 mg/dl and HDL is 50,

$$\text{cardiac risk ratio} = \frac{210}{50} = 4.2$$

See the box on the next page for a description of the risk profile common to many women with diabetes. Keep in mind that having these risk factors does not make you feel different or badly. That is why routine screening by your health care provider is important.

Get specific information about your own risk profile. Once you know your risks, you can learn to reduce them and prevent further problems. Use the grid on pg. 117 to keep track of your risk profile.

Common Risk Profile for Women with Type 2 Diabetes

Diabetes
High blood pressure: greater than 130/85
Abnormal blood fats:
    Low HDL, less than 40 mg/dl
    High triglycerides
    High cholesterol
Weight gain around the waist: having an apple-shaped body
    instead of a pear-shaped body
Sedentary lifestyle

Common Risk Profile for Women with Type 1 Diabetes
Diabetes

Taking action

Start reducing your individual risk today! To have the greatest impact, it is important for a woman with diabetes to stop smoking and get her blood pressure under control. Healthy life practices like yoga and meditation combined with a healthy lifestyle of activity and good nutrition are sure ways of strengthening your heart and blood vessels. Fiber is important in reducing cholesterol and triglycerides. Exercise increases muscle, which in turn reduces the blood fat and blood sugar levels. More muscle means more calories burned, even when you're resting!

Silly Bones: Osteoporosis

As a woman ages, her bones tend to become weaker, putting her at risk for a condition called osteoporosis. The conditions that pro-

Tests or Evaluations	Target for General Diabetes Population	Your Target	Your Current Levels
Smoking	None		
Activity level	20–40 minutes 3 or 4 days a week		
Meal plan	Low saturated fat, high fiber		
Blood pressure	130/85		
Triglycerides (fasting only)	Less than 130		
Total cholesterol	Less than 200		
LDL cholesterol	Less than 130 if no heart disease, Less than 100 if you already have heart disease		
Cardiac risk ratio	Less than 3.5 for women Less than 4.5 for men		

mote developing osteoporosis were set long ago by the food choices and lifestyle habits you made as an adolescent. Yet, there are things you can do today to protect your bones now. We would like to help you understand how having diabetes and being a woman puts you at risk for developing osteoporosis. Use the information in this section as a guide to discussing your risks with your health care provider.

Osteoporosis, which means "porous bone," is a condition in which bone mass is lost as a result of losing minerals and protein. Bones become very fragile and fracture easily. This condition usually develops slowly and after menopause. Estrogen, calcium, and vitamin D are important to the health and strength of your bones. Even though all women lose a little bone mass, not all women are at risk for osteoporosis. Some men develop osteoporosis, too.

Some women have characteristics that put them at risk for developing osteoporosis. These characteristics include:

Factors that interfere with the absorption of essential nutrients
• smoking

Body types associated with weaker bones
• fair-skinned women
• thin women, especially with limited muscle mass

Poor intake of the nutrients that build and maintain bone strength
• not enough total calories
• not enough calcium (particularly during pre- and early adolescence when bone density is at its peak)
• history of bulimia and anorexia

Health states that increase the risk for losing bone mass
• early menopause
• long-term steroid therapy
• prolonged high blood sugar (especially in type 1 diabetes)
• insulin deficiency (the bone loses mass and over time, becomes fragile)

Calcium is absorbed and deposited into the bone, which helps the bone to be strong and grow. A diet low in calcium, high in alcohol and caffeine, or a diet very low in fat weakens the bone. A little bit of fat is needed for the body to make estrogen, which is needed for building bone and preventing bone loss. Women with anorexia or bulimia must pay special attention to supplementing their diet with minerals, vitamins, and possibly HRT. If you have been caught up in the lose-weight-quick diet fads, have a history of eating disorders, or take in a very low fat diet, your bones may not have received the nutrients they needed to stay strong.

Body weight and muscle creates resistance, which strengthens the bone and promotes growth. Because most women with type 2 diabetes are overweight, they are less likely to develop osteoporosis. However, this is not true if your blood sugar is always high. Weight-bearing exercise is the best way to increase muscle mass and to protect your bone.

Preventing and treating osteoporosis

Every effort should be made to prevent excess bone loss and to keep bones as strong as possible. No matter what age you are now or how weak your bones are, you will want to pay attention to the suggestions below.

- Engage in weight-bearing exercise that helps to increase bone mass and density. Exercise should vary. Your body will respond nicely to exercise that involves repetition and muscle strengthening of the large muscle groups, including the quadriceps, hamstrings, abdomen, and back muscles. Even lifting small weights of one or two pounds helps increase bone mass and muscle strength.
- Stop smoking! Smoking interferes with calcium absorption and leaves the bones fragile and thin. Smoking is also a risk because smokers tend to eat a high-fat diet, drink excess alcohol and/or exercise less—all risk factors for developing osteoporosis.
- Eat a balanced meal plan that has enough calcium, phosphorous, and vitamin D. Ask a dietitian how you can increase these minerals in your diet.

- Get your diabetes under control!
- Consider HRT or other medications (Calcitonin, Fosamax) especially if you are at high risk or post menopausal. Explore this option with your doctor after reviewing the considerations below.

Hormone Replacement Therapy

Hormone replacement therapy (HRT) is the buzzword and therapy of the 1990s. Yet, there is a great deal of confusion about who is appropriate for HRT and how to take it. HRT has many potential benefits as well as risks. You and your doctor will want to determine whether it is appropriate for you, after careful consideration of your health and the possibility of developing side effects.

Advantages of estrogen

Estrogen itself is a female hormone that helps to keep the heart healthy and bones strong. It helps promote strong bones because it enhances vitamin D absorption, which in turn helps the body to use calcium effectively. Without estrogen, bone is more likely to weaken, especially if a woman is not active.

Many studies have shown that a woman can reduce her risk for heart disease by 50% if she takes HRT. It is believed that estrogen

- increases the body's production of HDL, the good cholesterol,
- decreases the body's production of LDL, the bad cholesterol,
- helps eliminate fat from the bloodstream,
- increases the blood flow throughout the body, and
- helps keep the blood vessels flexible.

Disadvantages of estrogen

Estrogen does have side effects. Taking high doses of estrogen is associated with an increased chance of breast and uterine cancer. Estrogen gives the body a "grow and divide" message. The uterus or breast tissue is sensitive to this message. If a woman has her uterus, she will need to take progestin to oppose the effects of estrogen. Progestin stops the "grow and divide" message and reduces the risk for developing uterine cancer.

In the past, oral contraceptives contained high doses of estrogen, which often interfered with the anticlotting factors in the blood. The blood clots more easily, putting the woman at risk for a stroke. In low doses, 0.625 mg or less, this is not a problem. The chance for stroke is higher in women with high blood pressure and who smoke.

A summary of the benefits and risks of HRT is listed in the box below.

Benefits of HRT

- Reduces bone loss during and after menopause
- Reduces symptoms of menopause
- Reduces the risk for heart disease by 40–50%
- Reduces wasting away of the vaginal tissue and discomfort

Risks When Estrogen is Taken Alone

- In large doses over long periods of time, increased risk for breast cancer
- If taken without progestin, increased risk for uterine cancer and bleeding
- Can make high blood pressure worse
- High doses may cause blood clotting problems

How HRT is used

The most important thing to remember is to work with a health care provider who knows the latest research and who is willing to discuss and not dictate to you. You have the right to seek other opinions. Most women will take HRT to protect them against osteoporosis and heart disease and to alleviate symptoms of menopause.

Before starting hormone therapy, it is important for you to have a thorough exam including a breast exam, pelvic exam and Pap smear; blood work that checks your liver function, thyroid function, cholesterol and triglyceride levels, calcium levels, and blood sugar; a mammography; and a complete family history, especially for breast and uterine cancer.

Here are some general guidelines to use when trying to understand HRT:

- Hormone therapy works for some women and doesn't work for others.
- Hormone therapy can cause extremely high triglycerides.
- Side effects from progestin, used in combination with estrogen, can cause women to feel anxious, depressed, or edgy.

There are three different ways of taking estrogen replacement therapy: oral estrogen, vaginal estrogen cream, and transdermal estrogen.

- Oral estrogen can be taken with or without progestin.
- Vaginal cream is effective for treating the vagina and urethra and is used to help treat menopausal symptoms that affect the female genitals. It has no effect on glycemic control. It is not effective for preventing osteoporosis.
- Estraderm, or the patch, does not increase the HDL cholesterol but does decrease LDL levels.

Osteoporosis
- Oral estrogen therapy is very helpful in preventing or halting the progression of bone loss.
- Vaginal creams or topical patches are not helpful in preventing osteoporosis.
- Supplements of calcium and vitamin D are important. Calcium intake of 1,000 mg per day is recommended.

- The combination of estrogen and progestin will also decrease the risk for osteoporosis.

Menopause
- Hot flashes and other symptoms felt during menopause can be reduced with estrogen therapy.
- Sometimes the dose is not enough to eliminate all the symptoms experienced during menopause. It is important to remember that the major goal of estrogen therapy during menopause is to reduce your risk for osteoporosis.

Breast and uterine cancer
- Estrogen should be given in the smallest dose possible to avoid the risk of cancer. The daily dose of estrogen should not exceed 0.625 mg/day.
- Estrogen gives the body a "grow and divide" message. When taken alone, it can cause the uterus to thicken and can eventually lead to uterine cancer and fibroids.
- Progestin gives a message that stops the "grow and divide" message. Therefore, it reduces the risk of cancer.
- Estrogen therapy is not appropriate for women with a personal or family history of breast or uterine cancer.
- If a woman has a uterus, she must take estrogen with progestin to reduce the risk of uterine cancer.
- If she does not have a uterus, she can take estrogen therapy without progestin, such as Estradiol, Estraderm, or Premarin.

Heart disease
- Estrogen therapy may reduce your risk for heart disease.
- Estrogen and progestin together may cancel out the benefit for heart disease but still help reduce the risk for osteoporosis.
- Estrogen therapy is not appropriate for women with a history of severe clotting disorder. The use of the transdermal patch or vaginal cream does not tend to affect the body's clotting ability and may be a treatment option.

How HRT Is Used

Estrogen Alone

- Protects against heart disease and osteoporosis
- Helps reduce symptoms experienced during menopause
- Not appropriate for women with history of breast or uterine cancer or of clotting disorders

Estrogen and Progestin Therapy

- Must be used if you have your uterus
- May not offer protection against heart disease
- Effective in decreasing risk of osteoporosis and symptoms of menopause

---

Taking Charge of Your Health

Remember, take one step at a time. Pick one risk factor to work on at a time. Exercise your rights and take charge of your care. Ask questions, check options, and do not make decisions before you feel comfortable. Ask for help and avoid isolation. Get professional help if emotional and physical distress wears you down.

Resources

For more information about women's health issues, see the following books. They are excellent resources and provide you with detailed discussions about the health issues described in this chapter. You should be able to find them in a library or book store in the women's health or health improvement sections.

Heart disease

Woman and Heart Disease. Edward B. Diethrich, MD, and Carol Cohan, Ballantine Books, New York, 1994.

Women, Take Heart. Richard H. Helfant, MD, G. P. Putnam's Sons, New York, 1993.

Overall health

New Passages: Mapping Your Life Across Time. Gail Sheehy, Random House, New York, 1995.

Women's Bodies, Women's Wisdom: Creating Physical and Emotional Health and Healing. Christiane Northrup, MD, Bantam Books, New York, 1994.

The New Our Bodies, Ourselves. The Boston Women's Health Book Collective, Simon and Schuster, Inc, New York, 1984.

The Diabetic Woman. Lois Jovanovic, MD, June Biermann, Barbara Toohey, Jeremy P. Tarcher, Inc, Los Angeles, 1987.

Anatomy of the Spirit. Caroline Myss, Harmony Books, New York, 1996.

Menopause

Menopause: All Your Questions Answered. Raymond G. Brunett, MD, Contemporary Books, Inc, Chicago, 1987.

Menopause, Naturally: Preparing for the Second Half of Life. Sadja Greenwood, MD, Volcano House, Volcano, California, 1992.

Menopausal Years: The Wise Woman Way. Susun S. Weed, Ash Tree Publishing, New York, 1992.

Hormone replacement therapy

Estrogen. Lila E. Nachtigall, MD, and Joan Rattner Heilman, Harper Perennial, New York, 1991.

Pregnancy

Diabetes and Pregnancy: What to Expect. American Diabetes Association, Alexandria, Virginia, 1996.

Gestational Diabetes: What to Expect. American Diabetes Association, Alexandria, Virginia, 1997.

Chapter 7

Problem-Solving: Real Women With Real Issues

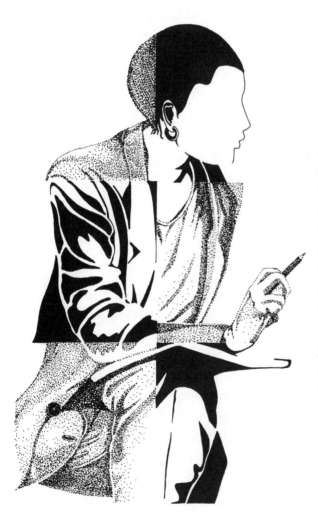

*Do not seek for the answers that cannot be given,
For you would not be able to live them and the point is to live everything.
Live the questions now and perhaps without knowing it, you will move along someday into the answers.*
—Catherine Feste

All women go through times when they do not honor themselves and their spirit. Whatever the reasons, emotional and physical health suffer as a result. Over time, a woman may come to realize that her choices, attitudes, and behaviors are not helpful to her. At these times, her inner wisdom can guide her to a healthier state. By listening to the messages sent by her body, she will gain the insight to change and regain her honor.

Some women realize this early in life, some later. Sometimes this awareness comes suddenly, causing you to make drastic changes in your self-care, relationships, or career choices. For other women, the realization is more gradual. However it happens, this insight does not remain constant. It has peaks and valleys. You get busy or forget, and you need to become aware again. It is over time that you gain a deeper appreciation of what is best for you.

When life gets hectic, it is difficult to stay in touch with your inner knowledge or to act in your best interest. Life presents many challenges. Are you choosing the path you follow? Or are you being pulled here and there by events? Are you developing your own signature, your own style of being? The stories in this chapter may help you become more aware of the choices you've already made and reveal other choices that you can make, if you wish.

> *It is never too late to embrace wellness of spirit and*
> *   mind.*
> *The body may not follow, but that is OK, for it is*
> *   only a cloak.*
> *Seek now to expose your inner healer and wise soul*
> *   that will guide you to a healthier state of being.*
> —Laurinda Poirier

In this chapter, you meet four women who, at different times in their lives, made decisions, developed attitudes, or engaged in behaviors that did not serve them well. Two women have type 1 diabetes and two have type 2 diabetes. Two are single, two are married, one has grandchildren. Their stories are about the dilemmas and choices involved in a woman's career with diabetes.

It isn't important whether or not they take insulin or have the same type of diabetes that you do. Listen to their internal struggles. How did their choices affect their self-care and feelings of well-being? These stories may make you realize things about yourself and the impact of your choices. Be kind to yourself as this happens. No matter what choices you made in the past, do not judge them. Look at your life with a new sense of hope. Witness the career paths these other woman have followed. What can you learn about listening to your own inner wisdom?

Lucy

Remember Lucy from Chapter 2? She is 48 years old and has had type 1 diabetes for 11 years. She is single and maintains a career as a graphic artist. Work and social commitments keep her very busy. Her diabetes-care program involves taking three shots of insulin a day (regular and NPH at breakfast, regular at supper and NPH at bedtime), checking blood sugar one to four times a day, and counting carbohydrates. She is committed to following an exercise program as a form of relaxation as well as for glucose management. This has not always been the case. Over the years her ability and willingness to pay attention to her physical and emotional needs were overwhelmed by competing priorities and events.

Periodically situations arise that challenge a woman's acceptance of her diabetes. Lucy reflects on some of her own personal challenges with accepting diabetes.

> *Traveling for my job is difficult. Occasionally I have to fly across time zones. This does such a number on my blood sugars, and I end up feeling horrible. I can't seem to manage my blood sugar levels as well as usual or exercise as often. And the food! I am either relying on airline food or eating in restaurants. Diabetes can be such a hassle. I resent having it!*

I am just beginning to deal with menopause. Up until seven months ago, I thought that I had come to terms with dealing with diabetes. I was able to manage the routine; you know, treat the high and low blood sugar and take my insulin on time. Besides that, I have just realized that because I have diabetes, my chances for developing heart disease is even greater! My father and uncle died of heart attacks in their early sixties! I get anxious knowing that I am getting closer to that age. I have to pay closer attention to my blood fats and fit exercise in! Sometimes I wonder, why me?

Having to confront her mortality and the potential for more health problems has Lucy feeling vulnerable, scared, and resentful. The positive thing is that she isn't running away from it. She's exercising more and getting her health care provider's help to bring the blood fat levels down. Her feelings are valid and honest. Her fear is real. And she isn't alone. Menopause forces every woman to stop and reflect on what her life is about. Diabetes has increased her risk for many health problems. It has also motivated her to do something about it. She can do things to help prevent heart problems from developing. What she needs to do to take care of her diabetes is often the same thing she needs to care for herself in general.

A woman's attitude about diabetes often changes from the attitude she had at diagnosis.

When I was first diagnosed, I had just lost a young nephew in an accident and my brother was diagnosed with cancer. When they told me that I had diabetes, I thought that it was manageable. I thought of it as an inconvenience but felt confident that I could figure out what and when to eat, and take the medication the correct way. But now, things are different. I dealt with it better then than I do now. When I realized that diabetes was going to last forever and the early symptoms of complications appeared, I began to feel how much freedom I had lost. Recently, my doctor told me that my kidneys were spilling small amounts of protein. Yikes! I wanted to take care of it right then. Then the eye doctor told me that I had small dot hemorrhages in my eyes. I was, and still am, so frightened and angry that I have diabetes.

Facing complications, Lucy felt fear, panic, and bewilderment. She had worked hard to take care of herself. She felt that meant she was not supposed to have problems. The body is complex. Many factors contribute to physical health. It is important to remember two things. First, she was able to prevent these problems from developing earlier because she took care of herself. Second, she had them diagnosed early. This is the time when treatment is most effective. She and her health care provider can keep an eye on these problems and prevent them from getting worse. Her emotions are a normal response to a crisis. However, Lucy needs to take control of her emotions so they do not control her. You can deal with any challenge that comes up in your life if you believe you can, and reach out for professional support.

Sometimes your treatment program just won't work for you. Working women need to be able to fit the treatment regimen into their work schedule. Not all jobs or employers allow you to take time out to eat or check blood sugar.

When asked what part of the treatment plan did not fit, Lucy identified the need to check her blood sugar and take insulin before lunch. It was difficult to get a break before lunch or find privacy, so she could not check her blood sugar or conveniently take insulin.

You need to see how the tasks involved with your diabetes care will fit into your daily schedule. If you are on a treatment program that requires you to check your blood sugar, draw up your insulin dose, or eat certain foods, you need to feel comfortable doing it in front of other people or arranging the time to do it elsewhere. If the treatment program doesn't fit, you won't be able to follow it and may feel guilty or frustrated.

Diabetes challenges women financially: Diabetes expenses will affect all the other events and circumstances in your life.

> *I balance my expenses for diabetes care supplies with the money I put aside for my rent, food, and other such expenses; for going out with friends; and for retirement. I am thinking about buying a house or condominium. I would love my own place! Last year things got tight because my car broke down. I needed to buy another one. That was an unexpected expense. I found myself cutting back on glucose testing. Sometimes I panic thinking what will happen if I could not work or if my health failed. I really feel the pressure to stay in my job, especially for the health benefits.*

For Lucy, having a steady income and having access to health care are real concerns. Lucy must prioritize how she spends her limited income and deal with the need to buy insulin, strips, and other self-care supplies. She could give up other things she wants for the things that she needs.

To manage life with diabetes you must deal with other people, their perceptions about you and your choices, and your own expectations for perfection.

> *People have so many misconceptions about my actions and my diabetes! Whatever I put in my mouth seems to be monitored by other people. I can't tell you how many times I hear "Are you supposed to eat that? Be careful, you might get complications." How am I supposed to feel after that?*
>
> *You know, sometimes I tell people that I am low as an excuse to eat something "sinful!" Otherwise I*

have to deal with a barrage of opinions, arguments, or questions. At those times I get defensive. I already feel guilty. They just reinforce what I already know. It is like putting salt in the wound. It isn't as if I don't want to do what is right; I just don't do everything perfectly all the time. It makes me feel like a little girl again!

I was brought up to be a good girl. To be a good girl and have diabetes means to have good HbA$_{1c}$ levels; not to cheat on my diet; and to exercise as often as I should. There are times that I don't do what I should, and I feel guilty.

Lucy understands that other people's comments are expressions of caring, but they still make her feel bad. It is tricky not to feel attacked. The challenge is to listen, to think about what is meaningful, and to let go of the rest. She feels caught in a bind of "shoulds." This drives her to make hasty decisions and to judge her own actions and choices harshly. When she realizes this, she can change the way she feels and thinks.

A woman's relationship to diabetes is often colored by weight and food. She can feel constantly assaulted by an "ideal" image of what she should look like.

I never seem satisfied with my weight. Because I am short, I feel I should also be petite. But I am not. I am a size 12 when I want to be a size 6. My diabetes makes it harder. I know that better blood sugar control will mean that it is harder for me to lose weight or even keep my weight where it is. I also know that if I do not take care of my diabetes, I will feel lousy, my kidneys will fail, and I will go blind. I know that I will feel guilty and that other people are going to blame me if that happens. Sometimes I feel that I cannot win!

I get really angry that I have to eat when I don't want to. Like when I have to treat a low blood sugar or prevent one. I resent not being able to eat what I want when I want!

Diabetes treatment programs do set a certain schedule of eating and medication taking. Eating just to prevent low blood sugars can take away from the pleasure of eating. Lucy is also frustrated that her body shape doesn't match her desire to look the way she wants to. On one hand, she wants to lose weight, and on the other she wants to pay attention to her blood sugar. One seems to make it difficult to do the other. It seems easier to give up and not try. Her dilemma is familiar to many women with and without diabetes. Yet her goal of being a size 6 is unrealistic. Genetically she is not meant to be that size. Striving for this will always cause her emotional pain.

Lucy deserves a great deal of credit! After careful consideration of the pros and cons, she decided to focus on her diabetes control. She realizes that her physical and emotional well being are not going to improve if she ignores her diabetes. Lucy is now redefining her goals. She is focusing her attention on how to be fit, not thin. Instead of focusing her attention on feelings of deprivation, she is focusing them on what she is able to do. She is learning how to look at her body and to love what she sees. Giving it negative messages because of her weight is unhealthy and will lead to more internal stress, imbalance, and "dis"ease.

A variety of attitudes and circumstances disrupt a woman's ability to follow through with her intentions to take care of herself.

I get tired of it all the time. It is so monotonous and requires too much structure. Eat now, check blood sugar, take medication. I can't get away from the clock! Sometimes because of stress, hormones, hunger, or fatigue, I don't feel like exercising. Sometimes I get sick of it all!

Taking care of my diabetes takes time. I have to think about what I am going to eat, figure what my dose should be, and take time to check my blood sugar. I get tired of these tasks and having to take time out of my day that I don't want to give up. I do have other things to do!

Lucy "learned the ropes" about taking care of her diabetes long ago. Doing these tasks is second nature to her. The spark of newness or excitement is gone. Being bored with the routine interferes with her level of motivation. It is important that Lucy recognize her need for renewal and rejuvenation. She needs and deserves a break from the dull routines. She needs support dealing with the effects of hormones on her diabetes control, which further threatens her energy and commitment. Creating time away, a vacation of sorts, may help Lucy regain her enthusiasm. Learning a new strategy or discussing her ambivalence with a good listener helps.

Diabetes can affect the way a woman relates to others and how others relate to her.

I don't like to let people know that I have high blood sugar. They might automatically assume I did something I wasn't supposed to.

In the past, I was on steroids to treat a health problem. During that time, my blood sugar was very high! I was still new with diabetes and I didn't know exactly what to do. I was weepy and depressed and very tired. I felt insecure. Diabetes affected my personal relationships. I thought everyone was mad at me, I had no tolerance for anything. I know I exaggerated everything, but I was so angry and scared at myself. I felt out of control. I withdrew. I was so miserable that many people stayed away. I know if I could have shared these feelings, I wouldn't have felt alone.

*I now know who and when to call if my diabetes gets
out of control. I have also learned how to adjust my
insulin and carbohydrates. Now that I know how I
feel when my blood sugar gets this high, I do
something about it right away.*

The feeling of powerlessness over what is happening in your
body or emotions can be overwhelming. There are so many factors
that affect blood sugar control, such as medications, illness, and
major life events. For Lucy, taking steroids caused very high blood
sugar, which further drained her. The time when she wanted to
reach out and be hugged is the very time she overreacted and turned
people away. It takes confidence to say, "I am sad, I don't know
what to do. Please, could you help me?" Thinking she should be
in control all of the time interfered with Lucy's ability to ask for
help. She lost valuable support and compromised her well-being.

Lucy is single and has had the opportunity for several serious
relationships. She has concerns about revealing that she has diabetes as well as about the prospective partner's ability to relate to
and understand her needs.

*It is difficult enough to find a partner in life without
adding in "Diabetes 101." How and when do I say,
"Oh, by the way, I have diabetes?" When do I talk
about what diabetes would mean for a long-term
relationship? Sometimes it is just too difficult.
Diabetes is not easily explained. How do you discuss
with a potential husband that long-term complications
could be in your future? Is he willing to accept that
for better or for worse? Is he, given a choice, going
to live with diabetes?*

*Then there is me. So much of what has meaning in my
life has to do with diabetes. What would change if I
were to include a husband in my life? I guess I have
to keep doing what is important to me and believe that,*

if the right person comes along, diabetes may enhance
his life just as it has mine.

Diabetes brings many unforeseen challenges and opportunities. Some women feel comfortable sharing these challenges with another person. Others limit this opportunity. This choice depends on how you see yourself and diabetes. Lucy has a legitimate concern. A prospective partner must want to and be able to deal with real and potential problems. Just as it took time for her to learn how to deal with diabetes, it will take him some time, too. She needs to be patient and honest. Neither one of them can see into the future. An intimate relationship is built on flexibility and understanding.

Help and support come in different packages and from different people. Another universal theme for women is having difficulty letting others help or take care of them.

> *I am very fortunate to be surrounded by a wonderful support system of friends. As a single person, I do not have a significant other to share some of the responsibility of taking care of me, including taking care of my diabetes. Who, then, do I choose to inform what my dose is, where the glucagon is, and how to give it to me, just in case I need help? Even though I do not have one person, I do have many people who help me in varying degrees. For me it is also an issue of control. I don't want to be a burden—I can take care of myself just fine, thank you very much. I guess I treat sharing my diabetes like sharing anything else. I can take care of it. It would be a weakness if I didn't.*

There may not always be one special person to share the responsibilities of managing life or your diabetes. Lucy has built her support system to include friends and family who help fill her life and provide her with support. Lucy struggles with allowing someone to help her without feeling guilty. She feels ashamed because she can't do it all. Her expectations of being totally self-sufficient and not reaching out for support may not be in her best interest. It is OK to ask for help. It doesn't mean she is weak. We all need help from time to time.

Dreams of the future can provide motivation for taking care of yourself. Lucy can see herself as a healthy 68 year old, going to school, and learning new things. She loves children and hopes to help young people with diabetes.

> *I keep trying. When things don't go right and my blood sugar is all over the place, or my health is bad, I deal with it. I have found a wonderful doctor and diabetes educator who work with me. I also learn as much as I can. I'm no longer fooled by thinking that knowledge is enough. Knowledge doesn't take care of this disease. Behavior does. I have to change my behaviors if my health is going to be the best it can be.*

Being aware of your vision for the future is important. It will give you motivation when you need to keep going. Lucy has also made a valuable connection with a health care provider who works well with her. She feels heard and listened to. Knowing what is needed to be well isn't enough. You do have to apply what you know and change risky behaviors or negative attitudes into healthy and positive ones.

To live in a state of wellness with a chronic disease requires forgiveness—forgiving yourself for not being perfect, for making mistakes, for not giving it your best all of the time.

> *I have a hard time forgiving myself. I always think that I am never going to manage diabetes like I should. Other people can do it much better.*

Lucy is under the illusion that others manage their lives and diabetes perfectly and that she is the only one who doesn't. Her rational side tells her this isn't so, but her emotional side fears that she isn't trying hard enough.

No one can live perfectly with a chronic disease. Too many unpredictable events and circumstances affect glucose control, emotions, and body responses. This is the time to let go of the illusion that perfection is possible. Good managers know how important it is to be nonjudgmental and flexible in this job. Forgiving yourself is critical to your well-being. Women need to forgive themselves as they forgive others. Carrying a grudge and holding on to hurt or anger helps no one.

Hanna

You met Hanna in Chapter 3. She was diagnosed with type 1 diabetes when she was five years old. She is now the mother of two girls and works at a local school as a teacher aide. Currently she is going to school to become a special education teacher with a focus on hearing impaired students.

Let's look at Hanna a year ago. She was on the treadmill of life. She was trying to develop herself intellectually by taking two classes a week, to meet the needs of her husband, children, and house, and to fit diabetes care in wherever she could.

> *I was 15 pounds overweight. I had struggled to lose weight after having my children. I took insulin twice a day. However, on busy days I often forgot my shot and took it after breakfast and sometimes, hours after dinner. I checked my blood sugar when I felt funny and treated low blood sugar when it occurred. Otherwise, I didn't have the energy or take the time for self-care.*

She was and still is committed to being a good mother, wife, and companion. The needs of her family and home conflict at times with her need to go to school, do her homework, and do her job at the local school. Superwoman syndrome lurks in the background! She has not included herself on her list of priorities.

Maintaining friendships and letting people know about her diabetes was always an issue. She had so little time for friends and feared being judged by her peers.

> *I* *didn't have time to go out with my friends. I had forgotten what it was like having a heart to heart talk with a friend. I hadn't been out shopping or to the movies in ages. I didn't even have time to go on a date with my husband! I felt guilty because I didn't spend enough time with the kids. I didn't know who I was. I felt isolated and alone.*

Even though she was busy, surrounded by many people, she felt alone. Discouraged with her weight and unhappy with her overall look, Hanna had too many priorities to be fair to herself.

Hanna's health began to suffer, requiring her to stop, reflect, and develop a different approach.

> *I* *had frequent vaginal infections, was tired all the time, and cried at the drop of the hat. I was snapping all the time at my kids. School was more difficult. I knew my life was out of control when I became unconscious because of low blood sugar and required treatment in the emergency room. My grades suffered and my marriage was tense. My kids suffered the most. I was cranky when I was high and just plain irritable when I was low. I felt so bad.*

Hanna was disconnected from her body. She hadn't taken the time to notice what her body and spirit were telling her. She ignored the muscle aches and the messages that she was on overdrive. She just kept pushing and pushing until exhaustion and severe hypoglycemia slapped her in the face.

Today things have changed.

*I am learning how to take some time for me while still
caring for my family and going to school. I have had to
learn that I can share some of the responsibilities with
other people, and I don't have to do everything on my
own. I am learning about quality time with my family.
Now that they are older, it is a lot easier. Being a good
mom doesn't mean being with my kids all of the time. I
worked with a diabetes team who started me on three
shots of insulin. Surprisingly enough, it is easier because
I am less likely to have low blood sugar during the
middle of the night. I now check my blood sugar two to
four times a day for four days out of the week. I talk to
the nurse every two weeks. She helps me adjust my dose.
My kids even help remind me to take insulin. I even let
them stick my finger. I never thought about getting my
kids involved. The diabetes educator helped me figure
out how to include them. I think it's a good thing.*

*I also see a dietitian who is helping me to lose some
weight. I really haven't liked my body. I just didn't have
the energy to plan healthier meals. Eating on the run
was our life!*

Hanna was forced to realize that she had to organize and refocus to feel well. With support, she was able to identify how she
could share self-care responsibilities with her family. She is learning how to use the skills and talents of diabetes care professionals. It may not always be easy, but it is a healthy career decision!

Hanna's self-care program included much more than taking
insulin and checking blood sugar. She negotiated with her husband
to share some of the daily routines to give her some time to get out
with friends and to exercise.

*I now start the day by waking earlier to do my
"diabetes thing." I also mentally think about what I
need to do that day. My husband helps to get the kids*

ready for school two days during the week so that I can go for a walk with a friend in the morning. Together, he and I have divided the chores in the house. He is giving a lot. I really appreciate it. I have a little more energy to pay attention to us as a couple. We are beginning to have some time together again. We go out on a date about once every two weeks, grocery shopping! I have a friend watch the kids for two hours so that he and I can have time together. I also need to exercise more to help me lose weight. I have looked into taking karate classes. Now that would be different!

Sharing the tasks and responsibilities has enabled Hanna to conserve her energy and focus it on the most important parts of her life. Sharing has allowed her to protect her most valuable asset, herself. She is beginning to honor herself and to respect her needs. Following this path will take her a long way toward fulfilling her goals of being a good mother and wife and of staying well.

Finances are an added burden for most families, especially when there is a chronic disease. This and the added pressures of daily life continue to put a strain on Hanna's marriage. She and her husband need to explore how to communicate their concerns to each other.

The cost of diabetes supplies, medical bills, and taking classes is a burden. Our finances are drained by diabetes. I want to be a normal mom and to provide for my children. Sometimes I feel guilty diverting money away from doing something for them to do something for me.

I don't want to be a burden to my husband. He does so much.

Her husband admitted being afraid of her diabetes, wanting to help but feeling helpless. "I don't know

*what to do for her. If I could, I would take it away.
I don't dare to ask her how she feels or tell her that
I am concerned about her choices in eating because
she will think that I am a nag. I wish I knew what
to do."*

Sacrifices must always be made. This is difficult. Communicating honestly with a loved one can also be very difficult. It takes courage to admit that you can't do it all alone. It also takes courage for your husband to admit his concerns so as not to hurt you. Frank discussion between you and your partner depends on you. Take the risk and give someone you care about the chance to tell you how much they care. From time to time, you may need the help of a family counselor to help you over the rough spots.

Sometimes a woman has to modify her goals to stay emotionally and physically healthy. Taking two classes on top of everything else was more than she could handle. Hanna was forced to reconsider how much time to invest in school.

*I was forced to realize that I could not continue at
that pace. I loved going to school. It was stimulating.
I was meeting new people and it got me out of the
house. I didn't want to give it all up so I decided to
take one course per semester. I will take a summer
class.*

By cutting back, she is able to take time out for herself and still manage the responsibilities of her family. It may take her a little longer to get her degree, but she will be healthier.

Motivated by the fear of complications and of dying early, some women try to do it all at once. Hanna lost sight of living in the present.

*As a young child, before blood glucose monitoring
was available, I didn't expect to be able to reach my
life dreams. I was afraid that future complications*

would interfere with the length and quality of my life. I felt the need to accomplish everything yesterday because I didn't think I would be able to do what I wanted in life. In focusing on what might happen, I haven't taken care of myself. Now with a clear vision of what I want to happen, I am motivated to take care of myself. Seeing my children grow up is important to me. I want to be there for them. I want to celebrate the good times and share the tough times. I won't be any good if I keep up this pace.

Hanna is on the treadmill of life, caught up in the "what ifs." She fails to live in the present and misses out on the small miracles that happen around her every day. Putting energy into worry about the future jeopardizes her well-being today. Her concern for the future has been fed by statistics that say people with diabetes die earlier than people without diabetes. These statistics were true in the past. With better tools for managing diabetes available, it is now possible for women to live long and fulfilling lives—but only if they pay attention to their needs today.

In her drive to do it all, Hanna lost sight of what was most important to her, her children and her husband. Continuing on the treadmill compromised her diabetes control and the relationships with her husband and children. She was not investing in the future.

Loretta

Loretta is a 72-year-old woman who has had type 2 diabetes for 12 years. She is married, with 5 children and 13 grandchildren. Originally she was taking diabetes pills. At the time of her diagnosis, she had high blood pressure and high blood fats.

Priorities in life change. Work, family, and friends can distract a women's attention from her self-care. Loretta's priorities today are different from the ones she had 12 years ago.

Getting diabetes was a blow. I now realize that I basically denied it for the first three years. Now that my blood sugar is lower, I feel better. I had no idea how bad I felt! For years, I loved to play bingo every week. This got me out of the house and gave me time with other people. I was busy with my family and work. It was exciting seeing my kids get married! At first I paid attention to the diet, but after a few months I started to cheat. I really love food, especially desserts. It was hard not to eat the way I used to. I never liked exercising, so I didn't walk like I should have. I didn't have the time to exercise, or so I led myself to believe! I didn't feel bad so I thought I was doing OK.

Twelve years ago, work, planning and cooking meals, doing the laundry, and cleaning house distracted her from paying attention to her diabetes and other risk factors. Take a moment to reflect on the words Loretta chooses to use—*diet* and *cheat*. As we mentioned before, words influence how we give meaning to things. Diet suggests depriving yourself of foods you like and only short-term weight loss. It isn't surprising that she only followed her diet for a short period of time. Meal plans bring guidelines for healthy eating into your everyday life, and you choose which foods to eat. It's a way of living and it's long-term. The meal plan is yours, the choices are yours, and your favorite foods can be included.

She was a devoted mother, helping her kids deal with life issues, and learning to be a grandmother. There were very few, if any, physical reminders of diabetes. It was easy to let self-care slip.

Uncontrolled diabetes, high blood pressure, and high cholesterol put Loretta at risk for problems with circulation.

Today I am on insulin twice a day. I am still 30 pounds overweight. I had two heart attacks and one stroke. After a lot of rehab I am pretty independent.

My husband is a great help. He is always asking me to go out for a walk. I am now retired so my day is not as hectic.

Loretta had many risk factors for heart disease. She did not appreciate how important it was to pay attention to her diabetes and blood pressure. This is common, especially when you don't feel bad. She did not realize how tired and sluggish she was. Today, she is working with her husband to improve her wellness.

Growing older has many blessings as well as losses.

Recently, my very close friend passed away. That has left me sad and scared. I was faced with the reality that I will die, too. For a while I began to question why I should bother with all this diabetes stuff. But then my granddaughter asked me to help her deal with a crisis. I felt honored to know that I was needed and that I could help. I then realized that I had a lot to live for. I know that I will die someday, but I don't have to rush it. There is a lot of living yet to do.

The nice thing about getting older is that I don't get caught up worrying about what other people think. I don't need to be perfect. In fact, I have learned to laugh at myself. I really do funny things sometimes!

Facing life and death is a part of getting older. It is magnified by having diabetes. You can live in fear of this and let life pass you by, or you can accept it and engage in life right now, every moment.

Loretta's wiser self allows her to enjoy her quirks. Taking life less seriously through laughter and a good sense of humor is an important tool to balance your perspective on life. Loretta has let go of the need for society's approval. She is comfortable being who she is.

Wellness is not defined by lack of illness or by physical health. It is an attitude. Loretta has a wonderful viewpoint on her current health.

I still consider myself healthy. I am able to say that I have high blood pressure, high cholesterol, and diabetes. I believe that if I am able to do for myself and to get out of bed every morning, I am healthy. I thank God that I can enjoy my kids and grandkids.

Loretta's attitude is very healthy and honoring! She is no longer denying that she has diabetes. It is a part of her to care for and nurture.

Small steps lead you forward to big changes.

I know that I need to eat less, and I try. I wish I would have made healthier food choices 5 and 10 years ago. Maybe I wouldn't have the problems I do today. When things get tough, I pick myself up and start all over again.

Change comes slowly. It isn't easy to change old behaviors. It is impossible to change what has happened in the past. Being realistic and less critical is an important step. No matter how small, each step takes you closer to your goal.

Every woman is motivated by something that she considers special. Sticking around to see her grandchildren grow up and get married is a real motivator for Loretta.

I want to see my grandkids get married! So I have to take better care of myself. Now I see a doctor regularly and respond to my needs promptly. I had a small problem with my eye, and I went to see the eye doctor right away. I didn't always do that.

When I am motivated or feel good about myself, I tend to exercise more. My husband is my coach. He doesn't let me get out of walking. He tells me that the dishes can wait until after we get back. I spend a lot of time with my children and grandkids. I love to go shopping with my daughter. That is a great diversion from eating.

I guess you could say that I keep a positive attitude, and...(pause) I try.

Loretta has faced many physical and emotional challenges. She has faced life-and-death issues. All of these trials and tribulations have helped her to stop and reflect on what is important in her life. This awareness drives her to get out and walk and to stop eating after she has had two small cookies. She has also learned to rely on her support people to help her. Being there for her grandchildren has given Loretta the reason to take better care of herself. This is infectious. Seeing her desire motivates her husband to be there for her.

She may not realize it, but Loretta is a successful manager of diabetes. She accepts her reality, practices self-care, and gets in touch with her sense of wellness every single day.

Dorothy

You met Dorothy in Chapter 3. She has type 2 diabetes, diagnosed at age 47. She is now 58, single, and a legal secretary for a law firm. She has had a long-standing relationship with a man five years younger than she. Two years before she was diagnosed, she was told that her blood sugar was a little high. She started a walking program that helped her bring her blood sugar down by the next time she went to see the doctor. She thought that she was OK.

The stage of life a woman is in, how she invests in herself, and the amount of energy she has can affect how she relates to her diabetes.

I was happy with my work and all that I managed to accomplish in my life. But I had reached a point that I wanted someone to take care of me. I was tired of taking care of myself. I wanted someone else to decide what to eat. Or to shop or cook without me having to ask. I would have loved for someone else to make decisions. I have no children to rely on. My parents were elderly at the time and not able to help me. Then I was diagnosed with diabetes. What a blow! It was one more thing that I needed to take care of.

Dorothy was responsible for managing her home, paying the bills, doing the cleaning and cooking as well as planning the social calendar. She was pleased about her working skills but wanted to share the responsibility for doing it all. Diabetes added to her sense of burden, demanding more attention and expenditure of energy.

Events in a woman's life challenge her ability to focus on her own self-care needs.

With the diagnosis, I began to watch what I ate. My job was very demanding, calling for extra hours over the weekend. This demand conflicted with my intentions to exercise and carry out my routine chores. For a while I watched what I ate and started walking again, but my job got in the way. Between taking care of my home, paying attention to my boyfriend, and working, I didn't take time to exercise. It was kind of easy to let exercise go because it isn't something I enjoy.

It is still a mystery to me why I don't do what I need to do. Even though I know better, I still don't follow the meal plan or exercise as I could or should.

Remember when Lucy learned that knowledge isn't everything? Well, Dorothy found that, too. Managing diabetes depends on her changing old habits in eating and exercising. Any attempt to make a change is important. However, to make lasting change a woman must truly want to do what is necessary. You have to break through your natural resistance to change the behavior or attitudes that sabotage your efforts.

It is also important for Dorothy to let her health care provider know when the treatment program isn't working for her. She may need more medication or to start on new therapy. The critical thing is not to let blood sugar stay out of control too long. By paying attention to her blood sugar levels and monitoring changes in how she feels, she can keep in touch with her diabetes and her body. Intentions to change behavior are great, but if unfulfilled, they don't do any good.

Some women feel skeptical about telling other people that they have diabetes.

> *I don't tell many people that I have diabetes. I don't want people watching what I eat or questioning why I am eating. My friend who knows about my diabetes will sometimes tell me that she is concerned when she sees me eating. I know that I can't eat any way I like. But some people assume that they have your best interest at heart when they say things. After all, I have the right to abuse my body if I want.*

> *There are times that I purposefully run my blood glucose levels a little high. I tend to guard myself by eating more than I need to in order to prevent a low blood sugar during a meeting at work. I know how to treat low blood sugar and all, I just don't want to deal with other people's responses if I do have one.*

Choosing to use the word *abuse* implies a feeling of worthlessness. It is linked with feelings of guilt and shame. She feels guilty about how she makes choices, even though she exerts a great deal of self control by eating a small bowl instead of the whole pint of ice cream. Using the word *treat* instead would acknowledge her power to make choices.

Dorothy is experiencing the emotional pressures of fitting diabetes into her life. Taking the time to learn to work with her meal plan helps. Dorothy is being realistic and practical about not going low during a meeting. If she takes care not to get too high by counting carbohydrates and checking her blood sugar before the meeting, she'll do even better.

Diabetes challenges women physically and emotionally.

Physically, I am challenged when I have high or low blood sugar. My energy is sapped, and I don't feel like doing anything. Low blood sugar interferes with my thinking ability and leaves me feeling incompetent. Actually, I can't follow discussions and lose my train of thought. My emotions depend on my physical functioning. When I try to do what I need to do for myself and it doesn't work, I get discouraged. The lack of success with the physical stuff influences my emotions. I try and think that I am in control. Things don't work out and I am left discouraged, thinking what am I to do?

The body, mind, and emotions are closely connected. More than the body is affected when your blood sugar goes haywire. Frustration easily rears its head. Many hidden factors influence glucose control, too. This may be a time to change your treatment strategy, soak in a hot bath, or go to the movies with a friend. Above all, don't forget to keep your sense of humor and to be kind and gentle with yourself.

Emotions affect how people feel about themselves and how much energy they have to take care of themselves. Dorothy found that when she felt good about herself, she was more likely do participate in self-care. When she was down, she didn't.

When I feel good about myself, I have enough energy to do what I need to do. I feel like I am being good to myself. That's nice. I don't even resent eating well! When I am feeling down, my energy is low. My blood sugar goes up because I don't feel like eating right or exercising. My mood gets worse, I feel even less motivated to care for myself, and I am more tired.

Depending on how I feel, I sometimes respond to the high blood sugar, sometimes I don't. I get very frustrated because my blood sugar bounces. It is a vicious cycle! I can't always get the sleep I need because I need to get up and take insulin. I need to spend some time problem-solving how to fit my diabetes treatment schedule into doing what I want to do. For example, sleeping in conflicts with taking my medication on time.

Self-care takes energy, patience, and time. In the best of times when a woman feels good and has energy, she can manage the crises or scheduling challenges. She does have the capability. However, it is a bit more difficult when she's fatigued, bogged down by high blood sugar, and feelings of helplessness. This is a good time to problem-solve other options with health care professionals or friends who can help her come to her own conclusions. Think of it as a friend helping you out of the fog on a path that you travel every day. We all need a little help sometimes.

Facing the facts about how she looks, her body, and her abilities takes courage! Not everything is in her power to change.

I struggle with knowing what healthy eating is and what my weight should be. I was 10 pounds lighter 6 years ago! It feels like food is on my mind all the time. I also don't have the look I want. I am never satisfied. Instead of losing, I gain. I don't have the energy to change the way I do things.

I still hate not being able to eat what I want. I am sad that I don't have the freedom. I can't go through a day without thinking about diabetes. Sometimes I think that I am going to get complications anyway. Most of my family did. So sometimes I wonder, "Why bother?" I know in my head that this is wrong, but in my heart, I am not so sure.

I use the pain from my finger stick to remind me that
I have diabetes and can't just eat anything that I want.
It is like a wake up call. I need these regular reminders.

For Dorothy, diabetes and her body are her reality. Looking truthfully at herself is very difficult. It is for many women. We might not like what we see. We may spend a lot of precious time trying to change something that cannot be changed. Remembering what is important in her life will help her face these truths and determine how she will define her sense of self. Dorothy courageously continues to face her truths.

Menopause can interfere with changes in blood sugar and overall energy. For some women, getting rid of the monthly cycles signals freedom. For others, it signals a loss of value and the nearness of death.

Over the last three months my blood sugar was acting very strange. Sometimes I have even had a low sugar—that is unusual for me! Other times, it is high and I am feeling crabby. This is all worse when I am stressed out about work. My doctor told me that it might be related to menopause. WOW. I guess there is nothing for me to do but accept it. I can't change my biological clock. This is very frustrating.

My symptoms of low blood sugar are very similar to having a hot flash. I now have to check my blood sugar when the symptoms occur to be sure which one it may be. It can be a hassle. My doctor and I are considering estrogen replacement therapy. My sister who is five years older than me told me that yoga helped her. I might try that as well.

Changes in hormone levels as a result of menopause can disrupt glucose control and make the body more sensitive to insulin. There are many options for dealing with the symptoms of menopause.

Patience and being gentle to herself during this time of transition is important. Remember, those HORMS!

Support from friends, health care professionals, and loved ones is needed for a woman to maintain integrity and a sense of balance in her career as a manager of diabetes and life.

I reach out to friends. Many are women or have diabetes. They allow me to share my struggles. That helps me realize that it isn't just me. I can unload. We give each other permission to be real and not perfect. I give them encouraging messages, and before you know it, I find myself listening to my own words of wisdom. They help me feel validated! I feel less guilty and that gives me a boost.

Women do not have to live with the pain of isolation or guilt. By sharing thoughts and experiences, you, too, can find that you are not alone. There may be no clear answer, but at least you know others share your struggles. Perhaps simply getting up each day and facing your challenges is the answer. It is certainly common to all human situations.

Getting Back on Track

During your life, you may find yourself straying away from your career path and your intentions of doing what is best for you. This is normal and happens to every woman. But if you are to experience wellness, you will need to reaffirm your intentions and to pay closer attention to your needs. It is possible at any age and during any point in your life to get back on track. Women can, and do, make changes in their lives. It is never too late to change your behavior or your attitude. Your life can be full and rich.

These women have learned to play an active role in their own lives and to respond to their physical and emotional needs. It has required them to learn about and respond to what their body needs, to forgive themselves for making mistakes, and to include themselves at the top of their list of priorities.

> *Our deepest fear is not that we are inadequate. Our deepest fear is that we are powerful beyond measure. It is our light, not our darkness, that most frightens us. We ask ourselves, Who am I to be brilliant, gorgeous, talented, fabulous? Actually, who are you not to be? You are a child of God. Your playing small doesn't serve the world. There's nothing enlightened about shrinking so that other people won't feel insecure around you. We are all meant to shine, as children do. We are born to make manifest the glory of God that is within us. It's not just in some of us; it's in everyone. And as we let our own light shine, we unconsciously give other people permission to do the same. As we are liberated from our own fear, our presence automatically liberates others.*
>
> —Marianne Williamson
> *A Return to Love*

Chapter 8

Life Practices That Matter

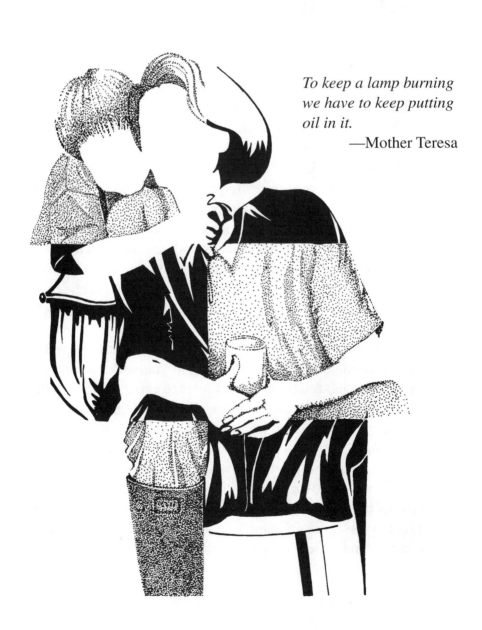

*To keep a lamp burning
we have to keep putting
oil in it.*
                    —Mother Teresa

Your career goal is to exercise your mind, your spirit, and your body to achieve wellness. You've got what it takes. We ask you to stop, listen, and realize what would nurture you at any given moment. Further, we ask you to think, feel, and act more optimistically. Listen to yourself today and over the next few weeks. Look for common themes or patterns. Realizing what you are actually doing can lead you to make some meaningful changes, just as realizing the patterns to your high blood sugar leads you to adjust your diabetes care habits.

Life Practices

What *practices* do you use to manage your health and your diabetes? We call them practices because you are practicing ways to care for yourself. The ways will change as you change. Practice is on-going, not something you achieve once and for all. Taking care of yourself is a process of meeting your needs by building on your own practices and adapting them to your current life circumstances. Your health care team, support groups, and diabetes literature can help you become aware of your needs and determine which practices to try. But you alone determine which practices will nurture you and how to fit each one into your life. Adopting practices that are right for you is the first step toward wellness. You are worthy of that.

Realizing what you need to do is one thing, but knowledge itself does not make the difference. Believing in yourself and changing your behavior does. You have already learned enough about healthy living to earn a PhD. Believe in yourself. Now is the time to commit the energy and make an investment in yourself.

It is common to try a new practice and give up. Generally, we try to do too many things at once and expect too much, too soon. As a result, we get frustrated and discouraged. Keep the following suggestions in mind as you adopt a new life practice.

1. Identify the area of your life you want to improve. Stop, breathe, and reflect on what is important to you right now.

2. Be realistic.

How can you do this? Pick one or two practices to try. Stick with them for several weeks.

3. Prioritize.

Commit the time and other resources necessary to adopt the practice. Don't give up, be persistent. You are in training, just like a new hire or an athlete.

4. Believe in yourself.

Fit this practice in with your existing lifestyle and make any necessary adjustments. Affirm your commitment by telling yourself that YOU CAN DO IT and YOU ARE WORTH THE EFFORT.

5. Expect challenges.

Your energy and commitment will go through peaks and valleys. Expect it. Your job is to prevent discouragement from affecting your ability to accomplish your goal. Seek assistance when you need it.

6. Enjoy.

It is exhilarating to accomplish a goal. Enjoy the rewards of the new practice. Build and use a support team to celebrate, and when necessary, motivate you.

Knowing what your goals are provides the motivation to develop and maintain healthy life practices. These goals also help you to get back on track when you are discouraged or bored. Everybody's goals are unique. To help you identify what your goals are, think about what you would like to be doing in 5 years and in 20 years. Use the list below to help you identify your own goals. Be careful not to choose too many at one time.

Worthy personal goals are
- to improve managing my diabetes
- to communicate my needs
- to nurture an intimate relationship
- to fulfill the needs once met by a relationship that has ended
- to nurture my children
- to prepare for a new venture (i.e., marriage, parenthood, retirement)

- to initiate or nurture a friendship
- to be fulfilled through volunteer work
- to be fulfilled through my hobbies
- to have fun
- to simplify my lifestyle
- to be fulfilled at work
- to experience sensual pleasure
- to enjoy companionship

Add your own goal

_____

Now that you have identified an area or two in your life that you would like to improve, ask yourself what you need to do to achieve your goal. The things you do will become the practices that help you achieve your vision for the future.

Take responsibility for yourself

> *Even though I may resist at first, I accept that only by being responsible to myself can I fully express my talents and experience the gifts of my life.*

Establish yourself as a priority. Before you can take responsibility for yourself, you need to promote yourself to the top of the priority list and give yourself the authority you need to take charge. Practice by taking over responsibilities for yourself in ways that you can manage right now. Learn to say no. It is OK. Learn to ask for assistance. It doesn't take away from your accomplishments or your commitment to others. Being "selfish" enough to take care of yourself and address your needs is healthy and a positive step toward wellness.

Be realistic. Make commitments that you *can* keep and follow through on them. The keys to doing this are *1)* set a goal, *2)* define at least four steps you can take to reach it, *3)* determine realistic ways to take each step, *4)* commit to your plan, *5)* follow through, *6)* celebrate your successes, and *7)* alter the plan as you see fit. Appreciate each small step you take. Achieving success, no matter how small, and building on it will demonstrate your abilities and build your self-esteem.

Communicate your needs. Be aware of what others can and cannot give you. Then remember that they cannot read your mind. State your needs. Be an advocate for yourself as a woman and a person with diabetes. This might feel strange at first, but advocating and speaking up for yourself is like lending support to a young child. There is no one more familiar with your personal needs and desires than you.

Ask questions until the answers are clear to you. Be aware of what others can and cannot give you. State your needs. Be clear about what you want. Practice saying what you want until you are confident that you are representing yourself well. You will find more resources than you thought. You are not alone.

Take calculated risks. Try new things. Join a group. Take a course. Ask a question. When you fall, pick yourself up and try again. Begin to play again. Or if you never played as a child, it's time to learn how. Play hopscotch, jump rope. Go hang-gliding or horseback riding. Take up piano or violin lessons. Build a model airplane and fly it. Have fun.

Quality living with diabetes in mind

I respect the daily challenges
that living with diabetes brings.

I honor my own wisdom and accept my own
limitations in meeting these challenges.

Trusting in my own wisdom and
the support of others, I can rise
to meet these challenges and thrive.

Find the help and information you need. To live comfortably with diabetes, you need to learn as much as you can about diabetes and your body. This is a lifelong learning process. Getting the information you need and finding adequate support while you are learning can be both rewarding and challenging. Spending time with other women who are at similar places on their career paths gives you information and support. People, publications, and the World Wide Web are all potential sources of useful support and information. You may feel pressured to learn everything all at once. Relax. Keep in mind that you can only absorb so much at one time. Remember that your emotions can easily cloud what you hear or read. Allow yourself to experience what is happening rather than forcing yourself to do things that you may not be ready for yet.

There are many wonderful diabetes programs and professionals to help you. Attending a diabetes education program is an important investment in your life and your well-being. It is worth the money you might have to pay! Below is a list of areas you want to be sure you know about. Use this list as a guide to determine whether you need to seek additional training and support.

Diabetes self-care skills

- Meal-planning strategies: how to plan your meals, count carbohydrates, and read food labels
- Activity guidelines: how to lead an active lifestyle and maintain body fitness
- Medication strategies: how and when to take medications so they work best for you
- Monitoring: how to check blood glucose, interpret, and respond to the numbers and patterns
- Hypoglycemia and hyperglycemia: how to detect, treat, and prevent them
- Sick day management: how to prevent life-threatening problems like ketoacidosis
- Foot, skin, and dental care
- Screening for complications: the tests to have and providers to see on a routine basis

- Guidelines for when to contact the health care team
- Ways to reduce your individual risk factors for getting complications.

Seeking the support of professionals

You have the right to work with a team of professionals who listen and respond to your needs. Recognize and respect the limitations of your health care provider. Prepare for your visit, write down questions that will help your provider focus on and address your concerns, and identify the areas that make it difficult for you to take care of your diabetes. Help your doctor treat you as a person. Report what is going on in your life that may be feeding or draining your energy and ability to follow your treatment program.

Diabetes professionals want to provide you with valuable information. They are also there to help you be a problem-solver and figure out how to make the diabetes program work for you. It takes time, patience, and fine-tuning to find out what works. Don't give up. They are your partners, and they need your active participation.

Practice regular renewal

*I deserve the time and quiet to
rejuvenate myself each day. Only in allowing myself
to focus can I be whole, happy, and healthy.*

You need practices to help you recover from the normal stresses of the day and to become more resilient for the bigger burdens you sometimes face. Stress, both physical and emotional, can be good for you as long as you have periods to recover. Recovery happens when you relax, gather your energies, and grow. You may be uncomfortable investing time and energy in yourself, but this investment pays big dividends! As a human being, you rebuild and recover through sleep, eating good food, laughing, and spending time with yourself in a pleasant, focused way. The attitude of work hard-play hard is a healthy attitude to adopt. Balance your energy. Be active. Be idle!

Here are some practices you could adopt to relax from your daily stresses and renew yourself for jumping back into your life.

Breathing. Your best friend is your breath. It is always there. Conscious breathing is the most powerful way to focus your energy inward and to relax. This is done by breathing deeply and rhythmically. You can practice this anywhere, at any time. With time and practice, you can develop the habit of responding to stressful situations with a calming breath instead of the more typical tightening up and shallow breathing. Practice getting in touch with your breathing by placing your hand on your belly. Breath into your belly, watching it rise as you inhale. Hold the breath far down in your abdomen for as long as you can. Let it out slowly and steadily for a count of 10. Relax and repeat. As you inhale, imagine bringing in warm air and sunshine. Exhale out any tension. Five minutes of abdominal breathing will give you lots of energy. Three such breaths in a tense situation can gather your forces quickly.

Create pause in your life. Slow your rhythm down to listen to your body and replenish your energy stores. Stop the treadmill from time to time. In Chapter 2, we speak about creating a vacation from some of your responsibilities. Discuss with a loved one or friend what others can do for or with you to give you some relief. There are things you can do for yourself. Always being busy does not have to interfere with your ability to experience the moment. For example, if you are washing the dishes, instead of thinking ahead to other things you have to do, try to focus on the moment. Enjoy the warmth of the water, a sense of accomplishment as the clean dishes mount up, the weight of your body balanced on the balls of your feet, taking slow, deep breaths. It is lovely to be alive in this moment; pay attention to it, and you'll have more energy for the next moment, too.

Relaxation. Relaxing is the art of doing what nurtures your body, slows down your mind, helps you ignore outside distractions, and focuses you inward. A hot bath, a nature walk, sitting with your cat, reading, doing yoga, drinking a cup of tea, listening to music, taking a jog, or walking the dog are all ways that you can unwind and relax. Practicing meditation in any of its many forms calms your mind and body into an elevated state of awareness. Achieving this state takes practice and commitment. You need to show up for your own renewal time each day. When you relax, you can be more aware of what is happening around you.

Rest. The average person requires six to ten hours of sleep a night. Doing what you can to ensure a good night's rest gives you an edge on the day ahead. Nighttime hypoglycemia can really foul up your night and your day. Work with your health care provider to resolve these sleep disturbances. Perhaps you need a snack at bedtime or to change your medication dosages. Sleep is a great and often overlooked healer. It can make the problems of the next day easier to face.

When you are tired, rest. Take a break during the day to recharge your batteries. Quiet your mind at the end of the day by relaxing with a hot bath, a good book, or meditation and set the stage for restful sleep. Make your resting place inviting and cozy. Watch your caffeine and alcohol intake before sleep. Think positive thoughts, and affirm your desire to gain perspective through sleep. Consciously clear your mind and relax your body. This daily practice is one of the most powerful ways to renew and rebuild your body and mind, yet little attention is paid to it. You perform best when you are relaxed and calm, when your energy is high, positive, and in control.

Take care of your body

My body is amazing. By taking care of any single part
of it, I am nurturing my entire body, mind, and spirit.

Honoring your body as it is right now. We are bombarded by messages to lose weight and fit into society's image of the ideal woman. If we focus on these external images, it is easy to think that something is wrong with our bodies. You honor your body through using it and listening to it. We must not accept the judgment of others to measure our own self-worth.

Healthy eating. Adopt a healthy attitude about eating. You can lose or maintain weight when you exercise and eat sensibly. People who exercise seldom gain back the weight they have lost. You are more likely to lose weight when you have muscle (it keeps on burning calories even at rest). Exercise helps you create muscle. When you diet, the first weight you lose is usually water. If you do not exercise, the next thing you lose is muscle. In addition, your metabolism slows down (as though you were going through a famine) and your body resists losing weight.

Food shapes who you are. It satisfies, rebuilds, energizes, and protects your body. It can also harm your body. Your food choices and eating patterns influence your energy level, blood-glucose control, weight, and even your resistance and susceptibility to some forms of cancer and heart disease. Our culture of fast food and fad diets has led us away from eating for nutrition. This makes eating for blood sugar control (and possibly weight loss) complicated. You need to be sure you are getting the nutrients you need and that you enjoy and feel nourished by what you eat. See a dietitian who will work with you on these goals.

Body works. It is important for you to get in touch with your body. Using the deep breathing and relaxation exercises described earlier is a place to start. In addition, give your body loving messages. Your body will respond in a positive way. Discard any critical messages. Andrew Weil in his book *Spontaneous Healing* suggests a practice for loving your body. First, identify one part of your body to work on, for instance, your belly. Second, stand in front of a mirror each day and focus on your belly. Speak to it directly, and tell it how much you love it. Tell it what you appreciate about it. "Belly, I love you." "I appreciate that you hold my essence." "Your shape is round and beautiful." Repeat these statements several times. Continue focusing on this part of your body for several weeks. Then move on to another part of your body.

Loosening up. Stretching, yoga, massage, and laughter release the tensions that accumulate over the day. These techniques can increase your strength, flexibility, and endurance. A well-toned and flexible body is better able to respond to physical and emotional stresses. If your body feels happy, your mind feels better, too.

Moving for recreation and fitness. Put some fun back into your life. Play! All children love to play. It is natural and a fun way to exercise. Movement can be referred to as fitness, exercise, play, or recreation. How you view what you do for movement can make the difference in whether you just endure it or truly enjoy it. Because your body, mind, and spirit are always connected, exercising your body will also invigorate the rest of you. However you choose to move your body each day, you will enhance the quality of your life and become more in tune with the real you. You will improve your diabetes, reduce stress, get better quality sleep, improve the way your body uses food, enhance your self-image, and reduce your risk of heart disease. Taking the initiative to exercise is a statement of your personal power and desire to be in charge of your own life. Sometimes this practice is difficult because of the pressure you put on yourself to do it right or to look just so. A simple thing like dancing or swaying to the music will open up new possibilities for enjoyment and flexibility. Relax and move in ways that feel comfortable. Remember to keep your spine in good alignment by imagining a string going out of the top of your head pulling you up into an easy balanced posture. Now breathe!

> *Why aren't you dancing for joy at this very moment?*
> —Pir Vilayet Khan, Sufi seer

Take care of your mind

> *I can gain mastery over my emotions and frustrations even though I may not be able to change the things that bother me.*
>
> *Clear thinking makes all of life's work easier.*

Keeping things straight. Diabetes brings a lot of equipment and tasks into your life. Life presents unpredictable challenges. Keeping things straight can really cut down on the time and stress related to having diabetes. Practices that help you get order are liberating. You have the time to do the things you want while taking care of the things you must.

Be mindful of the present. Focus on what you are doing. Pick one thing and give it your undivided attention. Make each moment count. Make it meaningful. You are creating memories.

Simplifying. Get rid of some of the tasks on your to-do list. Doing less while still meeting the challenges of life will give you more time to enjoy what life has to offer. Look at how you spend your time— keep a log if you need to—and consolidate or delete the things that are not necessary. Unclutter your life. Stop doing the things that you don't need or care about. Throw or give away things you don't use, such as clothes that don't fit. Plan several errands for one outing, like shopping for food when you go to get your hair cut or to the drug store. Whatever small steps you can take to simplify your life will bring you gifts of time and freedom.

Organizing. Make rituals for the things you do regularly. Keeping medication in the bathroom and taking it at the time that you brush your teeth makes it easier to remember. Being organized means you have a place for things and take the responsibility to put them back. It also means that you have thought through what you will need and have it available when you are ready. It is impressive how many creative ways people with diabetes have discovered to carry food, insulin, medication, and blood-testing equipment with them. Being organized is an investment in your future. For some people, this comes naturally; for others, it requires quite a lot of discipline and practice.

Quieting yourself. Solitude—being alone in relationship with yourself—is very different from being lonely. The difference is how you treat yourself in the relationship. If you listen, honor, and trust yourself, you will grow. This can sometimes be very uncomfortable.

If you have ignored, shut out, and distanced yourself from your own feelings, tuning into them now will require patience and support. Quieting yourself is an art. There are many practices that help you tune into yourself. These practices teach you ways to be calm and to put things into perspective.

Practicing yoga, meditation, and tai chi. These ancient practices provide a woman with the opportunity to tune into her body and quiet her mind at the same time. Deep breathing, centering, and stretching are key techniques used to focus the woman within. Consider learning from someone who has mastered them, someone who can be a mentor as you make these new practices part of your routine.

Be spontaneous. Learn how to pack your bag, change your meal plan, or adjust your diabetes medication so that you can be as spontaneous as possible and seize the opportunities that come your way.

Gaining sustenance from doing what you love. Fortunately, much of what women do is creative. This nourishes your heart and your spirit. Doing things that are creative and bring you gratification on a regular basis is one of the best ways to relax and relate to yourself. Gardening, ironing, cooking, dancing, reading, painting a picture, photographing nature, sewing, surfing the Net, or playing a musical instrument are all practices that can provide you with fulfillment. Many women find journal writing to be an effective means of connecting with their inner wisdom. Seek new ways to express who you are.

Taking care of your spirit

I can connect with my own spirit by reaching out to others, reaching in to my beliefs, and befriending my enemies, real and imagined.

This is how the practical brings you to the spiritual.

Feeding your soul

Balancing your time and energy. Balancing the time and energy you spend on meeting your responsibilities will lead to a more fulfilling life. Simply note how you divide your time between caring for yourself, caring for others, working, and playing. Distribute the time more evenly by focusing more on the areas that get less of your attention right now.

Schedule time in your day or week to do something that is good for you. This may be the time when you plan your healthy meals, exercise, or meditate. Taking care of yourself requires time, so protect it. Do not give it up even for a loved one. Imagine there is a fence surrounding this time with a gate that only you can open. When you are asked to fit something else in, close the gate.

Dealing with fear. Fear, like anger, is a normal emotion, but it is difficult to vent and release. While anger stimulates you to run or fight, fear often paralyzes you or hides behind other emotions. Avoiding your instinct to be afraid is not a good idea, but controlling your response to it can be. Fears common to women are: fears of failure, of rejection, of the unknown, of dying or isolation, and of loss of self control. Do you know what you fear? Trying to avoid those things you fear may result in decisions that cause you and others pain. Facing what you fear, although difficult, is always better because it forces you to develop a strategy and find out more about your own power. Facing what you fear is tough! Surrender and experience it. It will pass, and you will learn from it. You will see how strong you are.

Fear is very closely related to your level of self-esteem. When you are down on yourself, you are more vulnerable and sensitive to the things you worry about and feeling afraid is common. Building up your self-esteem does a lot to allay fear.

Allow yourself to heal. Let your tears flow. They promote healing, releasing emotions you can't express or recognize. Surrender and sit with the feelings. Listen to the insights and perspectives that arise from your own intuition. Share your story.

Write it down. Connect with a woman's group. When you need to, seek the help of a professional who can provide an objective perspective and help you unclutter the emotional chatter in your mind. Consider an attitude adjustment! Precious time and energy is lost being unhappy and focusing on things you cannot change. We need to focus on changing the things we can. Holding on to negative emotions is unhealthy.

Create more joy. Laugh. Let the spunky five-year-old girl who lives inside of you come out to play. Giggle, be silly, squish jello between your fingers. Open yourself to experiencing life with the freedom and innocence of this little girl. Look more often through her eyes. Each moment is new. Each event is special.

Befriending your enemies. "An enemy is always a teacher in disguise," says every wisdom teaching in the world. An enemy makes you uncomfortable and challenges your life practices, your beliefs, and your worldview. An enemy makes you change and possibly grow. You may discover new beliefs about yourself, learn new things, and develop new ways to relate to the people around you. The practices you've been following may be out of date. That's when you try on new ones and gradually replace the old ones to fit the person you want to be. Building on your new strengths and experience is the way to make changes that fit you. Work with, not against your own wisdom. Enemies can help you realize when you're fooling yourself. As you move up in your career, take time to look back at how much you have learned along the way.

Affirming what you believe. Affirmations are phrases you repeat to yourself throughout the day to reprogram how you view yourself and your life. This is positive self-talk. Just as an athlete develops muscle by practicing every day, you can develop your beliefs about yourself and your abilities. Your mind and spirit are like your muscle. To change a belief you need repetition, rehearsal, and practice, just as you do with building a muscle. You need to feed yourself with positive messages. Write down a short sentence that you can say to shift your thinking in the direction you want to go. For example, write "I communicate clearly" or "I am fun-loving." Write it on a piece of paper and put it where you will see it often. Read it several times each day, until it runs through your mind naturally. This practice helps make new practices, like meditation or exercise (play) fit into your conscious life.

Here are some more affirmations you can choose to repeat to yourself. Please create your own. You will soon see how positive statements of your own worth can be powerful tools to use.

- I am doing a great job!
- Boy, am I proud of the hard work I do to lose weight. Keep up the good work!
- I am amazing. I handle so much and balance so many things in my life that most women don't even think about once in their lives.
- I do a great job juggling the house, kids, school, and work.
- I love me for trying.
- I am a wonderful and capable person.
- I can make life decisions and be happy with them.
- I admire my strength in this new part of my life.
- I'm a great mom!
- My hard work has made a difference.
- I take care of my diabetes as well as I can.
- I make a refreshing difference in other people's lives.
- I forgive myself.
- My sense of humor is refreshing.
- When I am not in great control, I am not bad or wrong in my care techniques.
- I am OK just the way I am!
- All qualities exist in me. In each moment, I can choose the one I need.
- I am beautiful.

Each woman needs to remember the wisdom of her youth. Let's not forget what was clearer when we were so young.

> *I think I am very attractive. Who doesn't? Everyone is attractive, no matter what they look like. It's what is on the inside that counts, not on the outside. It's also your personality. I think that I am very unique and that is what makes me so special.*
> —Siobhan Perkins (age 12)

Recommended Reading

The Woman's Book of Courage: Meditations for Empowerment and Peace of Mind. Sue Patton Thoele, Conari Press, Berkeley, California, 1991.

Simple Abundance. Sarah Ban Breathnach, Time Warner, New York, 1995.

The Path of Love. Deepak Chopra, Harmony Books, New York, 1997.

Anatomy of the Spirit. Caroline Myss, Harmony Books, New York, 1996.

Spiritual Literacy: Reading the Sacred in Everyday Life. Frederic and Mary Ann Brussat, Scribner, New York, 1996.

The Women We Become. Ann Thomas, Prima Publishing, Rocklin, California, 1997.

The Art of the Possible. Alexandra Stoddard, Avon Books, New York, 1995.

NeuroSpeak. Robert Masters, Quest Books, Wheaton, Illinois, 1994.

Emulating Butterflies

As we move through the chaos, confusion, and
challenges of everyday life, we should remember we
have a winged and wonderful Self
within us, waiting to emerge from the darkness. Like
the butterfly, we need only go
into the stillness and solitude—to look within—to
find our wise Inner-Self waiting
to transform us through her knowing embrace.

Being gentle and patient with ourselves as we go
within is essential. Transformation takes time,
commitment, and discipline. Each day we need to
give ourselves the blessing of a few quiet minutes of
cocooning. We can have the courage to trust the
cocooning process and not expect
spectacular fireworks, or even insights at first.
It takes a while for our minds to become quiet
enough for us to hear the flutter of our inner wings.

—Sue Patton Thoele
The Woman's Book of Courage: Meditations
for Empowerment and Peace of Mind

Permissions

Struggle poem from *In The House of The Moon: Reclaiming the Feminine Spirit of Healing* by Jason Elia and Katharine Ketcham, Warner Books, copyright 1995. Originally published in *Quote* magazine, Las Cruces, New Mexico.

The Circle poem from *Spirit Walker* by Nancy Wood, copyright 1979. Reprinted by permission of Delacorte Press, Bantam Doubleday, Dell Publishing Group, Inc., New York.

Chart on pages 48–49 adapted and reprinted with permission from *Kicking Your Stress Habits,* copyright 1981, 1989. Donald A. Tubesing. Published by Whole Person Associates, Inc., 210 West Michigan, Duluth, Minnesota 55802-1908.

Virginia Satir quote from *Making Contact,* copyright 1976. Published by Celestial Arts, Berkeley, California.

List on pages 87–88 from *Self Actuated Healing* by Lonny J. Brown, copyright 1988. Reprinted by permission of Naturegraph Publishers, Happy Camp, California.

Quote from *A Return to Love* by Marianne Williamson, copyright 1992. Reprinted by permission of HarperCollins Publishers, Inc. Portions reprinted from *A Course in Miracles,* copyright 1975 by Foundation for Inner Peace, Inc.

Emulating Butterflies poem by Sue Patton Thoele reprinted from *The Woman's Book of Courage,* copyright 1996. Reprinted by permission of Conari Press, Berkeley, California.

Index

E

Eating out, 12
Education, diabetes, 162
Effective communication, 28, 51, 58, 62, 64–66, 69, 77, 103
Emergencies, 140
Emotions, 9, 17, 33, 46, 59–60, 69, 76, 80, 89–90, 96, 104, 110, 131, 136, 139, 151, 162, 167, 170–171
Employment, 21, 38
Energy, 5, 8–10, 12, 14, 20, 22–24, 29, 31–34, 40, 43–44, 49–51, 59, 61, 80, 91, 96–97, 100, 102–103, 135, 139, 141–142, 144, 148–149, 151–153, 158–159, 163–166, 170–171
Environment, 31, 96
Estrogen, 102, 105, 110–113, 118–125, 153
Estrogen replacement therapy (ERT), 112, 120
Exercise, 2, 10, 28, 34, 41–42, 47, 50–51, 54, 65, 67, 89–90, 92, 99, 103, 112, 116, 119, 124, 129–130, 133, 141–142, 145, 147, 149, 158, 166–167, 170, 172
  benefits of, 121
  blood sugar control and, 166
  guidelines for, 145, 163
  hypoglycemia and, 140, 162
  motivation, 41, 53, 58, 61, 135, 138, 159
  stress and, 6, 9, 25, 28, 52, 111–112, 134, 168
  tai chi, 169
  types of, 14, 16, 61
  weight loss and, 166
  weight training, 112
  yoga, 112, 116, 153, 164, 166, 169
Expectations, 6, 13, 21, 23, 42–43, 67, 96, 109–110, 132, 138
Eye disease, 9

F

Failures, 59, 132
Family members, 35
support from, 154
Fast-acting insulin, 76
Fast food, 166
Feedback, 29–31, 66–67
Feet, 37, 66, 81, 88, 164
Flexibility, coping with diabetes and, 5–6, 29, 71, 120, 139, 167
Food. See Nutrition
Food labels, 162
Friends, 10, 12, 22, 26–27, 30, 45–49, 59–60, 66, 72, 74–75, 77, 83, 85, 96, 110, 112, 114, 132, 137, 140–141, 144, 152, 154
  support, 5, 12, 20, 22–23, 25–26, 28, 30–32, 37, 44–45, 47, 56–64, 72–77, 90–92, 99, 135–138, 141, 148, 154, 158–159, 161–163, 169

G

Gestational diabetes, 125
Glucagon, 137
Glucose tablets, 109
Glycemic control, 29, 31, 110, 122
Grocery shopping, 142
Gum disease, 80–81, 132
Guilt, 5, 7, 10, 65, 82, 89, 91, 96, 150, 154

H

HbA$_{1c}$ levels, 105, 133
HDL cholesterol, 112, 115, 122
Health care providers, 11, 21, 25, 27–28, 32, 47, 60, 73, 76, 98, 108
Health care team, 12, 43, 72, 83, 91, 108–109, 158, 163
  access to, 132
  choosing, 25, 71, 90, 128, 150
  communication with, 73–74, 143
  doctors, 58
  dietitians, 25, 37, 73, 76, 107–108, 112, 119, 141, 166
  nurse educators, 37, 73, 99, 107
  physicians, 98
  questions for, 27, 124, 161
  team captain, 38